The GLP-1 Advantage
Beyond the Injections

Everything You Need to Know For Your GLP-1 Journey!

Written By: Brittany Alana

TABLE OF CONTENTS

(Page Numbers of Each Chapter)

04
Personal Introduction

11
Chapter One
Weight Loss Revolution

17
Chapter Two
How Semaglutide & Tirzepatide Work

24
Chapter Three
The Hormonal Connection

32
Chapter Four
Why GLP-1 Alone Isn't Enough

41
Chapter Five
Low Carb High Protein Approach

49
Chapter Six
Metabolic Benefits of High Protein

56
Chapter Seven
Breaking The Sugar Cycle

65
Chapter Eight
Why Sugar is the Enemy of Health

73
Chapter Nine
Weight Lifting & Resistance Training

80
Chapter Ten
Building Strength

89
Chapter Eleven
Preventing Plateaus

TABLE OF CONTENTS CONTINUED

96
Chapter Twelve
Beyond the Scale
Measuring True Success

104
Chapter Thirteen
Mindset Matters

112
Chapter Fourteen
Truth About Semaglutide
Face & Butt

122
Chapter Fifteen
Debunking Myths
Addressing Controversies

132
Chapter Sixteen
Side Effects &
Considerations

142
Chapter Seventeen
Hair Loss From
Rapid Weight Loss

149
Chapter Eighteen
Emotional Challenges
From Weight Loss

166
Chapter Nineteen
Societal Stigma
& Obesity

181
Chapter Twenty
Lessons Learned
From Challenges

188
Chapter
Twenty-One
Economic & Healthcare
Implications

193
Chapter Twenty-Two
Clinical Trials &
Evidence Based Outcomes

198
Conclusion

204
My Favorite
Recipes

INTRODUCTION

I want to say upfront, I'm not a doctor or medical professional... I'm simply sharing information I learned, through my own personal research, and from my own personal experiences along my journey. You should always consult with your own health care provider. With that disclaimer out of the way, who am I?

My name is Brittany Alana. I'm a 36 year old homeschooling mother of four children. They're my world, and as you can imagine, with four kids - I stay busy. So busy, that at some point, I started slacking on my health & self-care. I'm not making excuses. I take responsibility for how bad my weight & health got, but I think many moms in particular, can relate to what I mean! What little, "Me Time" I had --
I was exhausted & just wanted to chill.

It wasn't like I didn't try at certain points to lose weight. I can't tell you how many things I tried. Until I found one thing that worked, but I just had trouble staying on track. My weight kept yo-yoing, up & down like a roller-coaster, over the years, due to my struggle with...
Well, not cheating!

Until one day, unfortunately, I was diagnosed with type 2 diabetes. My labs also showed I had high cholesterol & high triglycerides. My blood pressure was bad. My weight had me medically listed as morbidly obese. And as if all this was not bad enough, I have a strong family history of heart attacks & heart disease on my mother's side -- Putting me at an extremely high risk!

My primary care provider and I discussed a plan for what to do, and she felt I was the perfect candidate for weekly Semaglutide injections. Later on, I then switched to Trizepaitide. Due to my health issues, my prescriptions were covered by my insurance.

I began my GLP-1 journey at 247 pounds. Fast forward almost a full year, and here I am, 102 pounds lighter, at 145 pounds! I've still got ten more stubborn pounds to shed before hitting my ultimate final goal. But man, isn't it amazing what can happen in a year?

My health has done a complete turnaround. Diabetes? Under control. Blood sugar? Stable. Cholesterol? Sitting pretty in the normal range. It wasn't just the numbers, though — I felt the change too.

More energy, better moods, and less huffing and puffing through basic tasks like cleaning the house. I no longer feel like I have to rush through taking a shower, because my weight made it hard to stand in a hot shower for long. I'd feel like I was gonna pass out, but not anymore! I can see my feet when Im standing up & looking straight down, for the first time since I was 20 years old.

So, how did GLP-1 injections play into all this? Well, they're incredible, but they're just one part of the equation. Let's clear up a common misconception:

While medicines like **Semaglutide and Tirzepatide** might sound like magic bullets, they're actually more like a powerful tool. But you've got to make use of your whole toolbox, with the other tools in that box; like good eating habits and regular exercise routines, to really see consistent progress and long-lasting success.

Sure, these meds help quiet that inner food chatter that can sabotage us, but they're not about to melt away those extra pounds, while we chill on the couch snacking away all throughout the day.

A lot of people will shame you, or belittle your success, as if GLP-1 shots are the easy way out. And hey, maybe you were hoping these shots would make the weight vanish without breaking a sweat.

But here's the real deal -- GLP-1s aren't a golden ticket to lounging away the pounds. They are not gonna melt the fat off for you, while you lazily refuse to make changes. Just because you're considering (or already using) meds, doesn't mean it'll all be smooth sailing from here on out. You've got to put in the work, by changing your eating habits and getting active. If you want steady, consistent, more effective weight loss, that stays lost for the long-term success... You can not stay on the same path that contributed to your obesity! That's just the reality of it.

Semaglutide & Tirzepatide are wonderful for silencing all the, "Food Noise," in your head. They help you fight temptation, and kick your carb addiction's butt...

I call it a **carb addiction**, not a food addiction, because lets be honest -- you were not craving veggies & meat! It was the carb-loaded stuff you wanted, that helped you become overweight!

These injections also slow down your digestion, so you feel full for longer. In other words, GLP-1s are great for keeping you on track. They reduce, if not eliminate, your urge to cheat & spiral out of control. It makes your healthier eating habits easier to stick to!
The rest, however, is still up to you!

Sure, you can lose a good chunk of weight in the beginning, just by not eating as much. You might think you can continue to eat unhealthy junk, as long as it's in moderation.

You'd be wrong.

At some point, your weight will stall & plateau; and regardless of what dosage your shots are, all progress will come to a halt. If your habits don't change, regardless of taking your shots, you'll begin to slowly regain your weight back...

We definitely don't want that to happen, right? Because then you'll feel defeated & stuck, for not seeing your weight go down, or for not reaching your health goals.

I've seen it firsthand with a family member who started Tirzepatide before me. After many months of progress, they stalled & hit a major plateaus because they didn't change their lifestyle. Even being on the highest dose did not help. I admire their initial success, and I'm rooting for them to get back on track.

But the lesson here? Use every stage effectively, by pairing it with healthy choices. Eventually, the meds' effects might fade a bit, and if you're already maxed out on dosage, like my family member is, where do you go from there?

They've reached the ceiling on dose adjustments and lost precious time, where changes could have brought them more success. Anyone can turn things around, with or without GLP-1's aid, but **starting smart** gives you the best shot... It gives you:

"THE GLP-1 ADVANTAGE"

Throughout this book, I'll be sharing everything I learned along my journey, to help guide you on your path. Learning from others' experiences can spare us a lot of time and trouble. I'm here to offer practical advice and genuine insight, not to sell you on a product.

This journey is about honesty, knowledge, and finding what works. I've packed in some yummy recipes and a weight loss tracking page, so you can grab a pen.

We're not alone on this adventure. Millions of people are considering, if not already taking, these weekly injections. I'm making this book, to help you, to the best of my ability. Let this book be another tool in your toolbox. You've got this!

It's your time to shine now. It's your time to succeed!

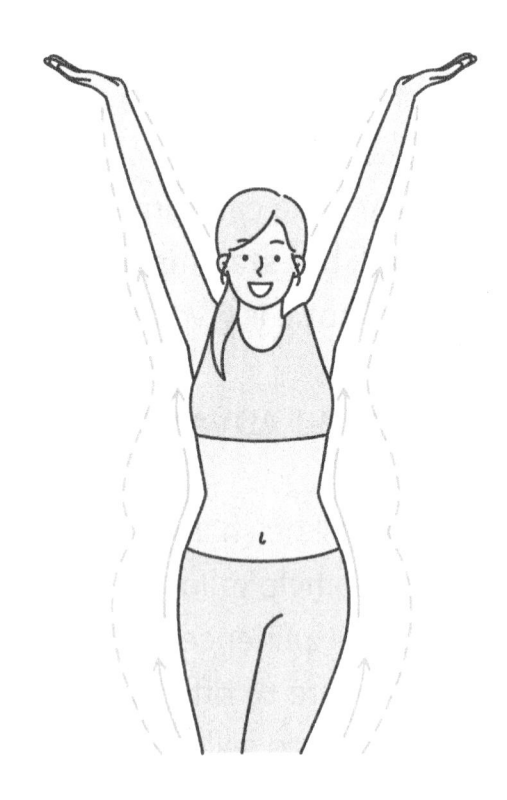

Chapter One
The Weight Loss Revolution

In recent years, a groundbreaking approach to weight loss has emerged that goes beyond traditional diet and exercise regimens.

At the heart of this revolution are GLP-1 (glucagon-like peptide-1) medications—namely, semaglutide and tirzepatide. These medications are transforming the way we approach weight management by targeting the body's hormonal pathways that regulate appetite, satiety, and metabolism.

This chapter introduces these innovative treatments and explores the science behind how they help regulate appetite and promote metabolic health.

Again, I am not a doctor, or medical professional. Just someone who did a lot of research along my journey, to learn this information for myself. Now I'm going to share it with you. Let's start with:

What Are GLP-1 Medications?

GLP-1 is a naturally occurring hormone produced in the intestines in response to food intake. It plays a crucial role in...

Regulating Appetite: GLP-1 signals the brain to reduce hunger and increase feelings of fullness.

Controlling Blood Sugar: It enhances insulin secretion in response to high blood sugar levels and suppresses the secretion of glucagon, a hormone that raises blood sugar.

Delaying Gastric Emptying: By slowing down the rate at which the stomach empties, GLP-1 helps prolong satiety and control food intake.

Semaglutide and tirzepatide are synthetic analogs designed to mimic —and in some cases, enhance— the natural effects of GLP-1.

They have been developed to provide a longer-lasting effect, making them suitable for weekly injections, as part of a comprehensive weight management plan.

These are not new medications, technically speaking. The first GLP-1 injections to be approved by the FDA, for the treatment of type 2 diabetes, has existed since 2005. Meaning there's tons of studies on how they impact the body, and what they are good for.

Despite the fact they were originally made for the treatment of type 2 diabetes, there's been enough evidence, through research & studies, to prove they are extremely successful at helping people lose weight.

They're still, to this day - 20 years later - conducting new studies and research, to learn more & more about these medications each day.

Never let anyone tell you, there's not enough information, to know whether or not these GLP-1 injections are safe.
There's 20 years -- and continuing -- worth of data!

The Science Behind Appetite Regulation and Metabolism
GLP-1's Role in the Gut-Brain Axis

One of the key innovations of GLP-1 medications is their impact on the gut-brain axis. When you eat, your intestines release GLP-1, which sends signals to the hypothalamus, the brain's appetite control center.

These signals do the following...
Reduce Hunger: They help decrease the desire to eat by increasing the sensation of fullness.
Modulate Reward Pathways: They affect the neural circuits that govern food reward, which can help reduce cravings, particularly for high-sugar and high-fat foods.

Metabolic Effects

Beyond appetite suppression, GLP-1 medications influence metabolism in several critical ways:

Enhanced Insulin Sensitivity: By stimulating insulin release when blood sugar levels rise, these medications help improve the body's response to insulin. This not only supports weight loss but also benefits overall metabolic health.
Reduced Glucagon Secretion: Lower glucagon levels contribute to more stable blood sugar levels, which is essential for reducing fat storage and promoting energy balance.
Delayed Gastric Emptying: This prolongs the time food stays in the stomach, leading to a slower absorption of nutrients. The result is a more controlled rise in blood sugar levels after eating, contributing to a prolonged sense of fullness.

Spotlight on Semaglutide and Tirzepatide

Semaglutide

Administration: Typically injected once per week. You can rotate between the 3 recommended injection sights of the body. Which are the fatty part of your stomach, the fatty part on the back of your arm, or a fatty part to the side of your thigh.

Mechanism: Mimics GLP-1 by binding to its receptors, enhancing insulin secretion and reducing appetite.

Benefits: Numerous studies have demonstrated significant weight loss, improved blood sugar control, and favorable changes in metabolic markers.

Tirzepatide

Administration: The same as Semaglutide. Once per week injection in one of the 3 recommended spots. Thigh, stomach, arm...

Dual Action: Unlike semaglutide, tirzepatide is a dual receptor agonist. A two-for-one deal! It not only activates the GLP-1 receptor but also targets the glucose-dependent insulinotropic polypeptide (GIP) receptor.

Enhanced Efficacy: This dual action may provide even greater benefits in terms of weight loss and metabolic control, offering a more comprehensive approach to managing obesity and type 2 diabetes.

Clinical Insights, via extensive testing & trials, have shown promising results. Such as the ability to help with sleep apnea, reduce risk of heart-related health issues, combat fatty liver disease, and the list seems to grow & go on as they do more studies...

It should be noted, that Tirzepatide is made by a completely different company, than the one who create semaglutide. While there is plenty of data over the last 20 years from the original versions, Trizepatide is sort of new to the scene, as far as brand & being a dual receptor agonist. The FDA first approved it in 2022.

The advent of GLP-1 medications like semaglutide and tirzepatide marks a significant milestone in the fight against obesity. By harnessing the body's own hormonal systems, these treatments offer a powerful tool to reduce appetite, improve metabolism, and ultimately support sustained weight loss. Especially, with combined with diet change & exercise!

Chapter Two
How Semaglutide & Tirzepatide Work

With all that in mind, I'd like to build upon the first chapter, by discussing the ways in which GLP-1 medications impact the body on a cellular & systematic level.

Call me a nerd, but I loved learning all the science of these injections while being on this journey. I'm putting these medications into my own body, afterall...
I wanted to know HOW they were functioning within me, on that type of level.

I feel we should always look up these sorts of things, and have a strong foundational understanding of what we are doing to our bodies.

I may not have always led a healthy lifestyle. I allowed my weight to get out of control at some point, but that doesn't mean I didn't care. I have always wanted to be healthy, and have tried to always be careful about what I put in my body.
So with that said...

Building on our understanding of GLP-1 and its role in appetite regulation, this chapter delves into the specific mechanisms of both semaglutide and tirzepatide.

By mimicking — or in the case of tirzepatide, enhancing — the natural effects of GLP-1, these drugs offer a powerful means to support weight loss and metabolic health.

Let's explore exactly how these two medications interact with the body, detail their modes of action, and explain the differences that set them apart.

The Mechanism of Action

Semaglutide

A Targeted Approach to GLP-1 Activation Semaglutide is designed to closely mimic the function of the natural GLP-1 hormone. Its key actions include:

Receptor Binding: Semaglutide binds to GLP-1 receptors found in various tissues, particularly in the pancreas and brain. This binding activates pathways that reduce appetite and stimulate insulin secretion when blood glucose levels are high.

Enhanced Insulin Secretion: When blood sugar rises, semaglutide promotes insulin release from the pancreas, which helps lower blood sugar levels efficiently. This is particularly beneficial for individuals with insulin resistance or type 2 diabetes.

Appetite Suppression: By sending signals to the brain's appetite centers, semaglutide helps reduce the urge to eat. This leads to a decrease in overall caloric intake, which is essential for weight loss.

Delayed Gastric Emptying: Semaglutide slows the rate at which food leaves the stomach, contributing to prolonged feelings of fullness and reduced food intake over time.

Tirzepatide

Dual Receptor Agonism for Enhanced Efficacy
Tirzepatide takes a slightly different, dual-action approach. Its mechanism of action includes:

Dual Receptor Activation: Tirzepatide activates both the GLP-1 receptor and the glucose-dependent insulinotropic polypeptide (GIP) receptor. This dual stimulation provides a more comprehensive metabolic effect.

Semaglutide usually ends with 2mg weekly as its highest dose. You hit this mark relatively quick, considering it does not go up as high as Trizepatide.

However, I lost the majority of my weight on semaglutide & was able to stay on 2mg for several months, before I ever transitioned to Tirzepatide's 5mg dose (which I'm currently on)

Clinical studies have demonstrated significant weight loss with both medications. Early evidence suggests that tirzepatide's dual mechanism might offer enhanced benefits for some individuals, particularly those with type 2 diabetes, though semaglutide remains a highly effective option.

Side Effects and Tolerability:
Common side effects for both medications include gastrointestinal symptoms such as nausea, constipation, or diarrhea. These effects often lessen over time, as the body adjusts to the medication. But it's important to work closely with your healthcare provider to manage these side effects and optimize the dosing regimen if necessary.

And as I mentioned in the introduction, there are ways to easily handle these side effects on your own, if you have any of them.

Feeling light-headed, or dizzy, when you first stand up is common, after you've lost a lot of weight & are on a higher dosage. This is usually your blood pressure needing a moment to "catch up" as you stand. Just give yourself a second, and it'll go away within seconds after standing.

Some people report having all-over body aches, like all the muscles in your entire body, all just had an intense workout, a day after taking your injection. It usually only lasts for one day. This also does not happen every time. I had this side effect only once, the very first time I ever took a GLP-1 injection. All I had to do, was just rest that day, let the whole-body soreness go away that day, and I've never had it happen again. Others say it only happens the first shot they take after titrating up in dosage.

Now, Im about to use a "Big Word," folks. Bare with me

...

Pharmacokinetics!

I told you I was going to be nerdy, and dish you all the scientific deets.

Pharmacokinetics is defined, "as the quantitative analysis of the processes of drug absorption, distribution, and elimination that determine the time course of drug action in response to an administered drug dose.

Pharmacodynamics deals with the mechanism of drug action." ... I'd say that's a pretty important thing to briefly touch base on!

The Role of Pharmacokinetics

Understanding the pharmacokinetics — the way the body absorbs, distributes, metabolizes, and excretes these drugs — is essential:

Long Half-Life: Both semaglutide and tirzepatide have been engineered to have an extended half-life, allowing for once-weekly dosing. This sustained release is critical for maintaining stable blood levels of the medication, ensuring continuous appetite suppression and metabolic benefits.

Steady-State Concentration: Achieving a steady-state concentration means that the body maintains a consistent level of the medication, which is key for long-term efficacy and minimizing fluctuations in appetite control.

In conclusion, Semaglutide and tirzepatide both represent significant advances in the fight against obesity and metabolic disorders.

By directly targeting the hormonal pathways that control appetite and metabolism, they offer a targeted and effective approach to weight loss.

However, as we will discuss in further chapters, their true potential is realized when integrated into a comprehensive program, that includes a balanced, low-carb, high-protein diet and a consistent exercise regimen. This holistic strategy is key to achieving lasting, sustainable weight loss and improved metabolic health.

Chapter Three
The Hormonal Connection – How GLP-1 Affects Your Body

Lets delve into the intricate network of hormones that govern appetite, metabolism, and energy balance, with a special focus on GLP-1.

Understanding how GLP-1 interacts with other hormonal systems in the body, is key to appreciating its role in weight management. From the gut-brain axis to its influence on insulin and glucagon, we need to explore the complex mechanisms by which GLP-1 shapes our eating behaviors and metabolic responses.

The Gut-Brain Axis: Communication at Its Finest
What Is the Gut-Brain Axis?

The gut-brain axis is a bidirectional communication system linking the gastrointestinal tract with the central nervous system.

This network allows the body to coordinate digestion, nutrient absorption, and energy regulation with cognitive and emotional responses.

GLP-1's Role in the Gut-Brain Dialogue...

Signal Transmission: After eating, the intestines release GLP-1, which travels to the brain to inform it that food has been ingested. This signal contributes to the sensation of fullness.

Appetite Modulation: By interacting with receptors in the hypothalamus—the brain's appetite control center—GLP-1 helps decrease hunger and curb food intake. This reduces the likelihood of overeating and supports caloric balance.

Neurotransmitter Interactions: GLP-1 influences neurotransmitter systems, including those related to reward and motivation. This modulation can lessen the appeal of high-calorie, palatable foods, thereby reinforcing healthier eating habits.

And it's that last one right there, ladies & gentlemen, Neurotransmitter Interactions that contribute to yet ANOTHER possible benefit these shots can be good for...
Fighting Addiction!

The companies that create these medications are currently conducting more research to further back this up. However, studies already done have shown this to be true...

And both my family member mentioned earlier, as well as myself, are proof that GLP-1s combat addiction.
Allow me to explain.

This family member of mine, smoked their entire life. Began smoking cigarettes when they were around 15 years old. Nothing ever made this person legit quit. They attempted to quit many times, but would cave-in easily & quickly, into each time they tried.

Being told they had COPD and had to be on an oxygen tank wasn't enough to make this family member quit smoking. Having a heart attack, needing triple-bypass open-heart surgery, and having heart disease was not enough for this person to quit ...

They knew they needed to, but were never able to do it successfully. Addiction is a pain-in-the-butt like that.

Until they were put on a GLP-1 and all of the sudden lost any desire to smoke.
At first, they assumed they were sick, and maybe that was why they were repulsed by the taste of cigarettes.
But nope...

Weeks turned into months... Months became almost 2 whole years now -- in their late 50's -- of not smoking anymore.

Which if this family member ever reads this book, I want them to know how I love them, and how proud of them, I am! Im glad they do not smoke anymore. I want them around for as long as possible.

For them, the addiction was cigarettes. For me it was carb-loaded food. I knew what I needed to do, what would work for me, to lose the weight. I could not resist my addiction to those types of foods. I would have a battle in my head that I lost to, every time there was something in the kitchen for my family to eat, that I wasn't supposed to have...

But when I began my shots? That battle in my head hasn't happened since! I couldn't care less what's in the kitchen for others to eat. I still eat, but I only eat when I need to now, and I can stay on track.

The sugary foods I loved before, taste horrible to me now; and make me feel sick at my stomach.

And because I have been without carb-loaded sugary foods for almost a whole year -- I can taste & enjoy the natural sweetness of certain foods and drinks, that most would think are not sweet at all!

It seems to be, that whatever you're addicted to, whatever you crave the most - and struggle to quit - these GLP-1s help silence it.

And understanding there's a **Neurotransmitter Interaction** that influence systems, like those related to reward and motivation, it now makes sense how & why!

Metabolic Harmony: GLP-1 and Insulin Regulation
Enhancing Insulin Secretion

One of the critical roles of GLP-1 is its ability to enhance insulin secretion in response to elevated blood sugar levels...

Glucose-Dependent Response: GLP-1 ensures that insulin is released when needed—specifically when blood glucose levels are high—thus preventing excessive insulin release when it isn't required.

Improved Glycemic Control: By fine-tuning the insulin response, GLP 1 contributes to stable blood sugar levels. This is particularly beneficial for individuals managing type 2 diabetes or insulin resistance.

Suppressing Glucagon

In addition to boosting insulin, GLP-1 suppresses the secretion of glucagon, a hormone that typically signals the liver to release stored glucose:

Balanced Energy Release: Lower glucagon levels help prevent unnecessary spikes in blood sugar, maintaining a smoother energy balance throughout the day.
Reduced Fat Storage: By stabilizing blood glucose, the body is less likely to convert excess sugar into fat, which supports weight loss and metabolic health.

Appetite Control and Satiety
Direct Effects on Hunger

GLP-1's actions extend to the brain's appetite centers, where it plays a pivotal role in regulating hunger...

Increased Satiety: The hormone signals when enough food has been consumed, promoting a lasting feeling of fullness after meals.

Delayed Gastric Emptying: By slowing down how quickly the stomach empties, GLP-1 prolongs the sensation of satiety. This delay in gastric emptying not only helps reduce overall caloric intake but also moderates post-meal blood sugar spikes.

Influence on Reward Pathways

Beyond physical signals of fullness, GLP-1 also affects the psychological aspects of eating...

Reduced Cravings: Its influence on brain regions associated with reward and pleasure helps diminish cravings for high-sugar and high fat foods.

Behavioral Impact: Over time, this can lead to a shift in eating habits, making it easier for individuals to choose healthier, more balanced meals.

Integrative Effects on Energy Balance
The Synergy of Hormonal Actions

The combined effects of GLP-1 on appetite suppression, insulin enhancement, and glucagon inhibition create a synergistic environment for weight loss...

Efficient Energy Utilization: With improved insulin sensitivity and balanced glucose levels, the body can more effectively utilize energy and reduce fat storage.
Support for Lifestyle Changes: By reducing hunger and moderating blood sugar levels, GLP-1 medications create a physiological environment that supports the adoption of healthier eating and exercise habits.

Long-Term Metabolic Benefits
Sustained Weight Loss: When GLP-1's hormonal benefits are paired with lifestyle modifications, the result is a powerful, sustainable approach to weight loss.
Overall Health Improvements: Beyond weight management, these hormonal adjustments can lead to better cardiovascular health, reduced inflammation, and an overall improvement in metabolic function.

The hormonal connection facilitated by GLP-1 is at the heart of its effectiveness as a weight loss tool. By bridging the communication between the gut and the brain, enhancing insulin secretion, suppressing glucagon, and moderating hunger signals, GLP-1 sets the stage for improved metabolic health and sustainable weight loss.

Chapter Four
Why GLP-1 Alone Isn't Enough

GLP-1 medications such as semaglutide and tirzepatide represent a major breakthrough in weight management, offering significant improvements in appetite regulation, blood sugar control, and overall metabolism. However, while these medications are powerful tools, they are not a standalone solution.

True, lasting weight loss and improved health require a comprehensive approach that integrates dietary changes, regular exercise, and sustainable lifestyle habits.

In this chapter, we'll explore why relying solely on GLP-1 injections is not good enough, and how combining them with dietary & lifestyle changes I made -- leads to superior, more long-term outcome.

The Limitations of Medication-Only Approaches
The Nature of Weight Loss

GLP-1 medications work by suppressing appetite and moderating blood sugar, but they do not fundamentally change lifestyle habits.

Once the medication is discontinued -- or is no longer working as effectively because your body got used to it -- without proper habit formation, there's a risk of reverting to old behaviors, leading to weight regain.

The body is adept at adapting to external interventions. Over time, the metabolic rate can adjust, and without supportive lifestyle changes, the efficacy of the medication may diminish.

Comprehensive Health Requires More Than a Pill (or Injection) Muscle Preservation:

While GLP-1 medications help reduce fat, they do not prevent muscle loss. Maintaining muscle mass is crucial for metabolic health and overall physical strength. Without the inclusion of resistance training and adequate protein intake, rapid weight loss can lead to a decrease in lean muscle tissue.

Nutritional Balance: Medications cannot replace the nutritional benefits of a well-balanced diet. The quality of the food you consume influences hormone levels, inflammation, and energy levels — all key factors in long term weight management.

Behavioral Factors: Psychological and behavioral habits around food and activity must be addressed for sustainable weight loss. Without developing healthier eating patterns and regular exercise routines, the initial benefits of GLP-1 injections may not be maintained.

The Role of Lifestyle Changes in Enhancing GLP-1 Benefits

Integrating a Low-Carb, High-Protein Diet

Optimizing Satiety: A low-carb, high-protein diet complements the GLP-1's appetite-suppressing effects, by promoting satiety (feeling full longer) and thus reducing your overall caloric intake.

Supporting Muscle Mass: Protein is essential for muscle repair and growth. Coupled with resistance training, it helps prevent the loss of lean muscle mass tissue, that can unfortunately accompany any form of rapid weight loss.

Stabilizing Blood Sugar: Reducing carbohydrate intake helps maintain stable blood sugar levels, further enhancing the metabolic benefits of GLP-1 medications.

They go hand-in-hand, like a match made in heaven. Ideal teamwork. This is especially the case for those suffering from any form of insulin resistance (for example those that have PCOS and/or Type 2 Diabetes struggle with severe insulin resistance) ...

Keep in mind, insulin resistance becomes a horrible vicious cycle that needs to be broken. If you are not responding to your insulin properly, the excess glucose is told to be stored away for a rainy day. Your body puts it in storage, aka FAT!

But because you are likely not as active as you need to be, and you eat regularly, you never tap into that storage. You never force your body to use up the fat it saved for future energy. And the more fat you have, the more insulin resistant you become.

Which leads to more glucose being told to go get stored away. You get fatter & more insulin resistant... A CYCLE! Which finally gets broken when you stop consuming the carbs that will become glucose in your body! You force your body to burn its fat!

The Importance of Regular Exercise

Incorporating weightlifting and resistance exercises is key to preserving and building muscle. This not only aids in maintaining a higher metabolic rate but also improves overall strength and functionality.

Cardiovascular Health: Aerobic exercise supports heart health and improves circulation, which is critical for overall well-being and for supporting the enhanced insulin sensitivity promoted by GLP-1 medications.

Combating Metabolic Slowdown: Regular physical activity helps counteract the natural metabolic slowdown that often accompanies weight loss, ensuring that the body continues to burn calories efficiently.

Building Sustainable Habits

Long-Term Behavior Change: Sustainable weight loss is achieved through gradual, lasting changes in behavior. This includes establishing regular eating routines, incorporating physical activity into daily life, and managing stress effectively.

Mindset and Motivation: Adopting a growth mindset, where challenges are seen as opportunities for learning and improvement, can lead to more resilient and sustained lifestyle changes.

Support Systems: Engaging with health professionals, nutritionists, fitness trainers, and supportive communities can provide the accountability and encouragement necessary for long-term success.

Building Sustainable Habits

Long-Term Behavior Change: Sustainable weight loss is achieved through gradual, lasting changes in behavior. This includes establishing regular eating routines, incorporating physical activity into daily life, and managing stress effectively.

Mindset and Motivation: Adopting a growth mindset, where challenges are seen as opportunities for learning and improvement, can lead to more resilient and sustained lifestyle changes.

Support Systems: Engaging with health professionals, nutritionists, fitness trainers, and supportive communities can provide the accountability and encouragement necessary for long-term success.

The Synergistic Effect: Medications Plus Lifestyle

Enhanced Efficacy: When GLP-1 medications are paired with a nutrient-dense diet and consistent exercise, the resulting synergy often leads to better weight loss outcomes and improved metabolic health.

Improved Adherence: Experiencing early success with medication can motivate individuals to adopt healthier habits. Conversely, a well structured lifestyle plan can reduce potential side effects of the medication and improve overall adherence.

Sustainable Results: The integration of GLP-1 treatments with lifestyle changes helps ensure that weight loss is not just a temporary fix but part of a permanent transformation in how you approach health and well-being.

Real-Life Success Stories

Case Studies: Numerous clinical studies and personal success stories illustrate how individuals who incorporate diet and exercise alongside GLP-1 injections achieve more significant and sustained results compared to those relying on medication alone.

Behavioral Reinforcement: Positive changes in energy levels, physical appearance, and overall health reinforce continued commitment to a healthier lifestyle, making it easier to maintain the benefits achieved during treatment.

I am living proof of this! I am sharing with you, the approach to weightloss I -- myself -- am using!
I have lost **102 pounds** so far.

You ever heard the phrase, "Don't just talk about it! Be about it!" ... Well, Im not just writing about it, I am all about the diet & exercise methods I suggest in this book.

And you can be a success story, too!
This book can give you information to consider & use, while you're on your own journey, if you want to.

GLP-1 medications offer a promising and effective tool for weight loss by targeting key metabolic and hormonal pathways.

However, without accompanying lifestyle changes — such as adopting a low-carb, high-protein diet, engaging in regular exercise, and developing sustainable healthy habits — the full potential of these medications cannot be realized.

This chapter emphasizes that successful and sustainable weight loss is not about quick fixes...

It is NOT taking an "easy way out"... but rather it's about building a foundation for lifelong health.

Chapter Five
The Low-Carb, High-Protein Approach

In the quest for sustainable weight loss, dietary choices play a pivotal role in complementing the metabolic benefits provided by GLP-1 medications. Among the various dietary strategies, a low-carbohydrate, high-protein approach has emerged as a particularly effective method. It's not the only method out there, but it is the only one that worked for me personally!

So we're going to explore why reducing carbohydrates supports weight loss and how increasing protein intake can enhance satiety and metabolism—laying the foundation for long-term success in your weight loss journey.

Why Reducing Carbohydrates Supports Weight Loss

1. Stabilizing Blood Sugar Levels
Reduced Insulin Spikes: Carbohydrates, especially refined sugars and starches, lead to rapid spikes in blood sugar, triggering large releases of insulin.

Insulin is a hormone that promotes fat storage, so frequent spikes can hinder weight loss efforts.

Enhanced Fat Burning: By lowering carbohydrate intake, you can minimize these insulin spikes, creating an environment where your body is more likely to utilize stored fat for energy.

2. Minimizing Caloric Intake

Lower Energy Density: Foods that are high in carbohydrates, particularly processed ones, often come with extra calories and lower nutritional value. Reducing these can help cut overall calorie consumption without sacrificing essential nutrients.

Improved Satiety Through Quality Foods: By focusing on nutrient dense foods rather than high-calorie, low-nutrient carbohydrate sources, you naturally decrease your calorie intake, which is crucial for weight loss.

3. Reduced Cravings and Appetite

Less Sugar, Fewer Cravings: A high intake of carbohydrates can lead to a cycle of sugar highs and lows, resulting in increased hunger and cravings for more sugary foods. A low-carb diet helps break this cycle.

Synergy with GLP-1 Medications: GLP-1 medications already work to suppress appetite and improve satiety. A diet low in carbohydrates reinforces these effects, making it easier to adhere to your meal plan and resist unhealthy snacks.

How Protein Helps with Satiety and Metabolism

1. Increased Satiety and Reduced Appetite

Long-Lasting Fullness: Protein is known for its ability to promote a strong feeling of fullness after meals. This satiety effect reduces overall hunger, leading to a lower total caloric intake throughout the day.

Hormonal Influence: Protein consumption stimulates the release of satiety hormones such as peptide YY (PYY) and reduces levels of ghrelin, the hormone responsible for hunger. This hormonal shift supports the appetite-suppressing effects of GLP-1 medications.

2. Enhanced Metabolic Rate

Thermic Effect of Food: Protein has a higher thermic effect compared to fats and carbohydrates. This means that your body burns more calories digesting protein than it does digesting other macronutrients, contributing to a higher overall metabolic rate.

Muscle Preservation and Growth: A high-protein diet, especially when paired with resistance training, helps maintain and build lean muscle mass. Muscle tissue burns more calories at rest compared to fat tissue, thereby boosting your resting metabolic rate.

3. Improved Body Composition
Maintaining Lean Muscle: Protein is critical for preserving muscle mass during weight loss. As you lose weight, ensuring adequate protein intake minimizes the loss of lean muscle, which is vital for sustaining a healthy metabolism.

Enhanced Recovery: For those engaging in regular exercise, particularly strength training, protein is essential for muscle repair and growth.
This not only aids in achieving a toned physique but also contributes to overall metabolic health.

Integrating the Low-Carb, High-Protein Approach into Your Lifestyle

Creating a Balanced Meal Plan
Prioritizing Whole Foods: Emphasize whole, unprocessed foods such as lean meats, fish, eggs, dairy, legumes, and a variety of low-carb vegetables.

These foods provide high-quality protein along with essential vitamins and minerals. You won't want to eat very much, so when you DO EAT, you want to make it count -- by being as nutritious as possible.

Smart Carb Choices: While the focus is on reducing carbohydrates, it's important to choose the right ones. Incorporate complex carbohydrates like leafy greens, broccoli, and other fibrous vegetables that offer nutritional benefits without spiking blood sugar. Fiber is a "Good Carb" and it is also your friend on a GLP-1 journey! You'll want some fiber each day, to help keep your bowel movements regular.

Timing and Portion Control

Meal Frequency: Consider smaller, more frequent meals to maintain steady energy levels and manage hunger. This approach can complement the slow-release nature of GLP-1 medications.

Or due to a lack of appetite, forcing yourself to eat frequently, even if it's small meals, might sound horrible.

So instead, focus on breakfast and dinner. Have your dinner be your biggest meal, between the hours of what normal lunch & dinner would be for you. So for example, if 7pm is my normal dinner time...

That's getting kind of late, I want my body to have more time to digest things before I go to bed that night, and I didnt have lunch! So I would have dinner around 4:30pm to 5pm, which is a little earlier. And it can be my last meal for the day, if I am no longer hungry.

Balanced Portions: Ensure each meal contains a balance of lean protein, healthy fats, and low-glycemic carbohydrates to support sustained energy release and muscle preservation.

Overcoming Challenges

Adapting to Change: Transitioning to a low-carb, high-protein diet may require an adjustment period. Plan your meals ahead of time and experiment with new recipes to keep your diet both enjoyable and sustainable. If you feel overwhelmed, or you just live a busy life, then keep it simple!

I know under normal circumstances I would have gotten tired of eggs, or my quick easy protein waffles... Or just throwing together a salad... I repeated my meals - and still do - so much that I should hate those foods at this point.

However, my relationship with food has changed since being on GLP-1s, and I personally no longer view food in the same way I once did before. Prior to GLP-1 injections, food was about comfort & enjoyment. Now? It no longer has that enticing appeal to it anymore. I still like food, Im just no longer in a mental space where it controls my thoughts. Im not living for food anymore. So keeping it simple & quick works for me! I can happily handle the repetition of foods I throw together, without getting sick of it. That sounds crazy, but it's honestly amazing.

I went from acting like an addict who was fighting with myself to maintain my "Junk food sobriety" -- and failing every time, eventually!
To now, just being like, "Meh!" (shrugs shoulders) "Dont need it. Im good!"

My shots help me to be okay with keeping it simple! Which prevents me from feeling overwhelmed by the dietary changes I made.

I now have free time, and space in my mind, to focus on other things, and new hobbies. Or even getting back into older hobbies, I'd stopped doing for a years. Like my love for writing!

Staying Consistent: Consistency is key. Combine your dietary changes with regular exercise and mindful eating practices, to create a lifestyle that supports long-term HABITS... The longer you do something & get used to it, The more it'll form it into a habit that'll feel more natural to you.

Adopting a low-carbohydrate, high-protein diet provides a strategic advantage in the journey toward sustainable weight loss.

Reducing carbohydrates stabilizes blood sugar levels, minimizes cravings, and limits unnecessary caloric intake; while a high-protein intake boosts satiety, enhances metabolic rate, and preserves lean muscle mass.

When integrated with GLP-1 medications, these dietary strategies work synergistically to create a comprehensive plan that supports long-term metabolic health and weight management.

Chapter Six
Metabolic Benefits of a High-Protein Diet

While reducing carbohydrates helps stabilize blood sugar and curb cravings, a high-protein diet does more than promote satiety — it also plays a critical role in boosting metabolism and preserving lean muscle mass tissue.

Let's explore how protein impacts metabolic rate, enhances energy expenditure through the thermic effect of food, and supports the body's adaptation during weight loss. Understanding these benefits is essential for creating a diet that not only helps shed pounds but also improves overall metabolic health.

Protein and Muscle Preservation
The Role of Muscle in Metabolism

Muscle as a Metabolic Engine: Muscle tissue burns more calories at rest than fat tissue. By preserving and even building muscle, you increase your basal metabolic rate, which means you're burning more calories even when not active.

Preventing Muscle Loss: During weight loss, there's often a risk of losing muscle along with fat. A high-protein diet supports muscle repair and growth, helping maintain lean mass and ensuring that the weight lost is primarily fat.

Benefits in the Context of GLP-1 Medications

Synergistic Support: GLP-1 medications assist with appetite control and metabolic regulation, but they do not prevent muscle loss on their own. Adequate protein intake ensures that the body has the building blocks necessary for muscle maintenance, complementing the benefits of the medication.

Enhanced Recovery: For those engaging in resistance training or weightlifting, protein aids in muscle recovery and adaptation, which is essential for sustaining long-term exercise habits that boost metabolism.

The Thermic Effect of Protein
Understanding the Thermic Effect

What Is the Thermic Effect? The thermic effect of food (TEF) refers to the amount of energy expended by the body in digesting, absorbing, and metabolizing nutrients. Protein has a higher TEF compared to carbohydrates and fats.

Calorie Burn Boost: Consuming protein increases energy expenditure because your body uses more calories to break down protein. This means that a high-protein meal not only provides the nutrients you need but also temporarily boosts your metabolism.

Practical Implications

Meal Planning: Incorporating protein-rich foods in every meal can lead to a cumulative increase in daily energy expenditure. Over time, this contributes to a higher overall metabolic rate.

Sustainable Energy: The increased thermic effect helps in creating a slight but consistent calorie deficit, which is beneficial for weight loss while still providing the necessary energy to fuel your day.

Protein's Role in Metabolic Adaptation

Supporting Weight Loss Without Metabolic Slowdown

Adaptive Thermogenesis: As you lose weight, your body tends to lower its metabolic rate as a defense mechanism against perceived starvation. A high-protein diet can counteract this effect by preserving muscle mass and keeping the metabolism active.

Hormonal Benefits: Protein intake supports the balance of hormones that regulate metabolism, including insulin and leptin. This hormonal balance is crucial for maintaining energy levels and ensuring that the body efficiently uses nutrients for fuel.

Long-Term Metabolic Health

Sustained Energy Levels: By preventing muscle loss and boosting metabolic rate, a high-protein diet helps maintain steady energy levels, which are essential for an active lifestyle.

Improved Body Composition: With a greater proportion of muscle relative to fat, your body becomes more efficient at burning calories, even during periods of rest. This improved body composition contributes to long-term weight management success.

Integrating High-Protein Foods Into Your Diet
Choosing Quality Protein Sources

Meats and Fish: Options like chicken, turkey, lean beef (such as 20/80 ground grassfed ground beef), and fatty fish (like salmon) provide high-quality protein along with essential nutrients like omega-3 fatty acids. Pork, such as bacon, ham, and "Pulled Pork" used for BBQ sandwiches...

Plant-Based Proteins: Legumes, tofu, tempeh, and quinoa offer excellent protein alternatives for those following a plant-based diet. I don't personally use tofu, but I wanted to add some plant options.

Nuts & Seeds: Almonds, walnuts, pecans, chia seeds, flax seeds, pumpkin seeds, pine nuts, hazelnuts, and "hemp hearts" are all examples of seeds & nuts that have healthy fats, fiber, and protein in them!

Dairy and Eggs: Greek yogurt, cottage cheese, cream cheese, and eggs are rich in protein and versatile for various meal preparations. Real Butter made from cream, Heavy Cream, and other cheeses (like cheddar or parmesan) have protein in them. However, moderation is key here. Use correct portion sizes, due to the fat content these dairy products contain.

Also, not all dairy is good on a low-carb lifestyle. Most yogurts nowadays, are loaded in sugar. Regular Milk used for cereals & so forth, is also high in sugar. Fake Butter made from oils is horrible for you. So just pay attention to the dairy you consume & be careful about which ones you're choosing!

Low-Carb, High-Protein does **NOT** mean you can never enjoy the foods you once loved. It just means replacing certain ingredients, and finding a new way to make those foods!

If you choose this type of diet, you will not go without, or feel deprived.

It's more likely to be very satiating. Mix that with the impact GLP-1 shots have on reducing your hunger, and you should be able to follow this style of eating without any regrets.

It's Easy-Peasy, Lemon-Squeezy, once you get used to it! I have recipes you can try in the back of this book.

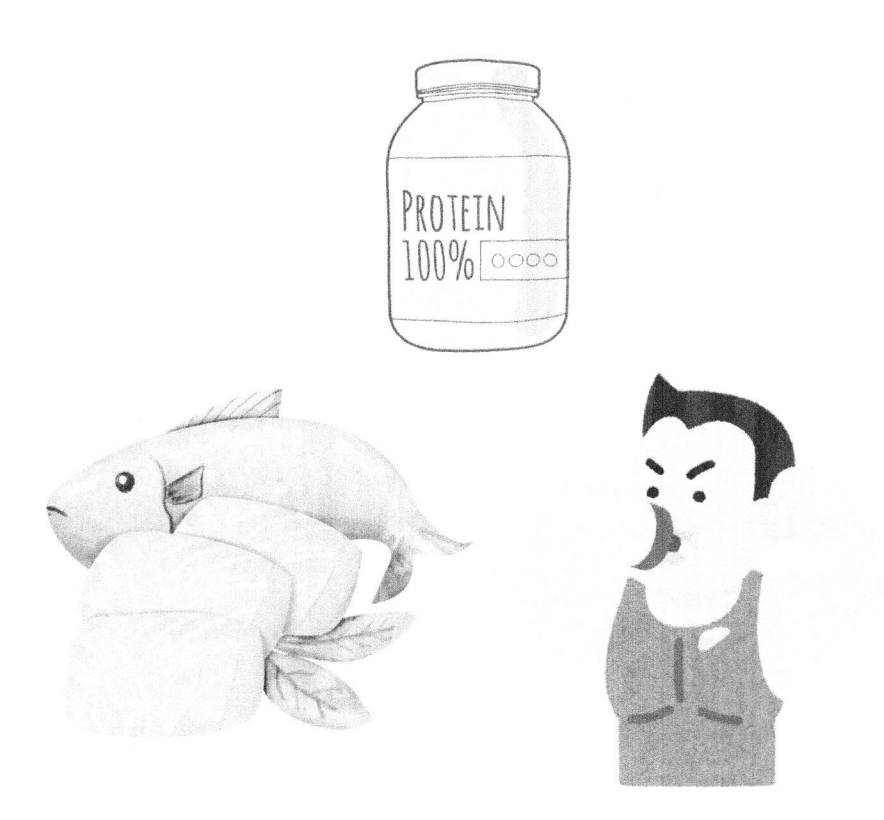

Chapter Seven
Breaking the Sugar Cycle

Regardless of what dietary plan you're wanting to follow... Even if you choose another method outside of Low-Carb & High Protein...

We have to get some FACTUAL things straight about Sugar, itself! It is so important to move forward on your journey, with a comprehensive understanding about sugar.

In today's food environment, sugar and highly processed carbohydrates are ubiquitous, playing a significant role in triggering cravings and promoting fat storage.

This chapter examines how these dietary components disrupt metabolic balance and create a vicious cycle of overconsumption, while also highlighting the stabilizing impact of GLP-1 medications on blood sugar levels.

By understanding these mechanisms, you can take proactive steps to break the sugar cycle.

How Sugar & Processed Carbs Affect Cravings & Fat Storage

1. The Rapid Rise and Fall of Blood Sugar

Insulin Spikes: Consuming sugar and processed carbohydrates leads to rapid increases in blood sugar. In response, the pancreas releases a surge of insulin to help cells absorb this sugar.

Subsequent Crash: The quick insulin spike is often followed by a rapid drop in blood sugar levels (a crash), which can trigger intense hunger and cravings for more sugar or refined carbs

2. The Vicious Cycle of Overeating

Cravings and Overconsumption: These fluctuations make it challenging to maintain steady energy levels. The body craves more sugar to regain energy, perpetuating a cycle of overconsumption.

Fat Storage: High insulin levels not only reduce the body's ability to burn fat but also signal the body to store excess energy as fat. Over time, this can lead to increased fat accumulation, especially in the abdominal region.

As I explained in an earlier chapter, body fat leads to insulin resistance, and being resistant to your insulin leads to more fat! you gotta break that cycle!

3. Impact on Metabolic Health

Insulin Resistance: Frequent spikes and crashes can lead to insulin resistance, where cells become less responsive to insulin. This condition not only hinders weight loss but also increases the risk of metabolic disorders such as type 2 diabetes.

Chronic Inflammation: High sugar intake is associated with chronic low-grade inflammation, further complicating weight loss efforts and overall health. This can lead to all sorts of health issues.

The Impact of GLP-1 on Blood Sugar Stabilization

1. Enhancing Insulin Sensitivity

Targeted Insulin Release: GLP-1 medications promote a more measured, glucose-dependent release of insulin. This means that insulin is secreted only when necessary, avoiding the excessive spikes that follow high sugar consumption.

Improved Blood Sugar Control: By ensuring that insulin is released in a controlled manner, these medications help stabilize blood sugar levels, reducing the risk of both spikes and crashes.

2. Reducing Cravings

Appetite Suppression: With more stable blood sugar levels, the intense hunger and cravings that typically follow a sugar crash are significantly reduced. This supports better portion control and healthier snacking choices.

Balanced Energy Levels: Consistent blood sugar levels help maintain energy throughout the day, making it easier to resist the lure of sugary snacks and processed carbs.

3. Breaking the Cycle

Empowering Lifestyle Changes: By stabilizing blood sugar, GLP-1 medications create an environment where healthier food choices become more sustainable. This allows for a gradual shift away from sugar dependency, fostering long-term dietary changes.

Synergistic Effects: When combined with a low-carb, high-protein diet, the benefits of GLP-1 are amplified. The dual approach not only curbs sugar cravings but also enhances overall metabolic function, making it a powerful strategy for sustainable weight loss.

Breaking the sugar cycle is a critical step in achieving lasting weight loss.
By understanding how sugar and processed carbohydrates fuel cravings and fat storage, and by leveraging the stabilizing effects of GLP-1 medications, you can disrupt this harmful cycle

Macros Can Matter – Finding the Right Balance

1. Understanding Macronutrients
Proteins: Essential for muscle repair, satiety, and a higher thermic effect, protein is a cornerstone of any weight loss plan, especially when combined with resistance training.

Fats: Healthy fats support hormone production, brain function, and the absorption of fat-soluble vitamins. They also provide a steady source of energy.

Carbohydrates: While often vilified, carbohydrates are an important energy source. The key is to choose complex, fiber-rich carbs over refined sugars and processed grains. Fiber is good! You want around 15g per day if possible.

(Hemps Hearts, Chia Seeds, and Flax Seeds are all good choices, that are a "Low Carb Diet Friendly" choice loaded in fiber. Your dark leafy greens, asparagus, and broccoli. Unsweetened Cocoa Nibs or Unsweetened Dark Chocolate. Almonds, hazelnuts, and walnuts help with fiber -- **to list a few ideas**)

1. Determining Your Macro Needs

Individual Factors: Your ideal macronutrient ratio will depend on factors such as age, gender, activity level, and specific health goals. Consulting with a nutrition professional can help tailor a plan to your needs.

General Guidelines: Many successful weight loss strategies emphasize a higher protein intake, moderate healthy fats, and a reduced intake of refined carbohydrates. Making sure that any carbs you do ingest are primarily Fiber.

An example, of what your diet ratio should look like, should be **60% protein, 35% fats, and 5% carbohydrates** — but an adjustment might be necessary based on your personal health, or for lifestyle reasons, at different points in time... If you've hit your goal weight, and you're now in "Maintenance Mode" -- your body wont have as much fat within its self to consume, and you will no longer be worried about muscle mass loss from rapid weight loss.

So in this case, you may want to adjust your macros to something that looks more like -- **50% Protein, 40% Fats, and 10% Carbs!** You can play around and tweak it as you see fit, as long as your carbohydrate intake never goes above that ten percent of your daily macros. And as long as they're primarily Fiber.
Remember Fiber is the only "Good Carb" on this diet...

Tracking and Adjusting: Utilize tools such as food diaries or digital apps to track your intake and adjust your ratios as needed. Regular monitoring allows you to fine-tune your diet to ensure you're meeting your energy needs while promoting fat loss.

Portion Control: Use this opportunity on GLP-1 injections to pay attention to portion sizes, to avoid consuming excess calories, even when they are considered "healthy foods." Even for foods that are good for you, it is possible to over eat.

However, being on these medications will help us feel full faster & for longer. Take advantage of that now, while you can.

Get acquainted with the portions you can tolerate, before feeling full. How much food was it? Learn to stop eating when you feel full. Listen to your body.

Those smaller portions you are eating, because you feel full faster, is the portion size it should have always been eating prior to your GLP-1 shots.

If for any reason, you have to stop taking semaglutide or trizepatide, you'll now be aware of what the smaller portions looked like, and formed a habit in only eating that amount.

By calculating the right protein, fat, and carbohydrate ratios, and structuring your meals to support sustained energy and satiety, you set the stage for long-term success.

Coupled with the benefits of GLP-1 medications and a low-carb, high protein approach, managing your macros effectively can empower you to achieve and maintain your weight loss goals.

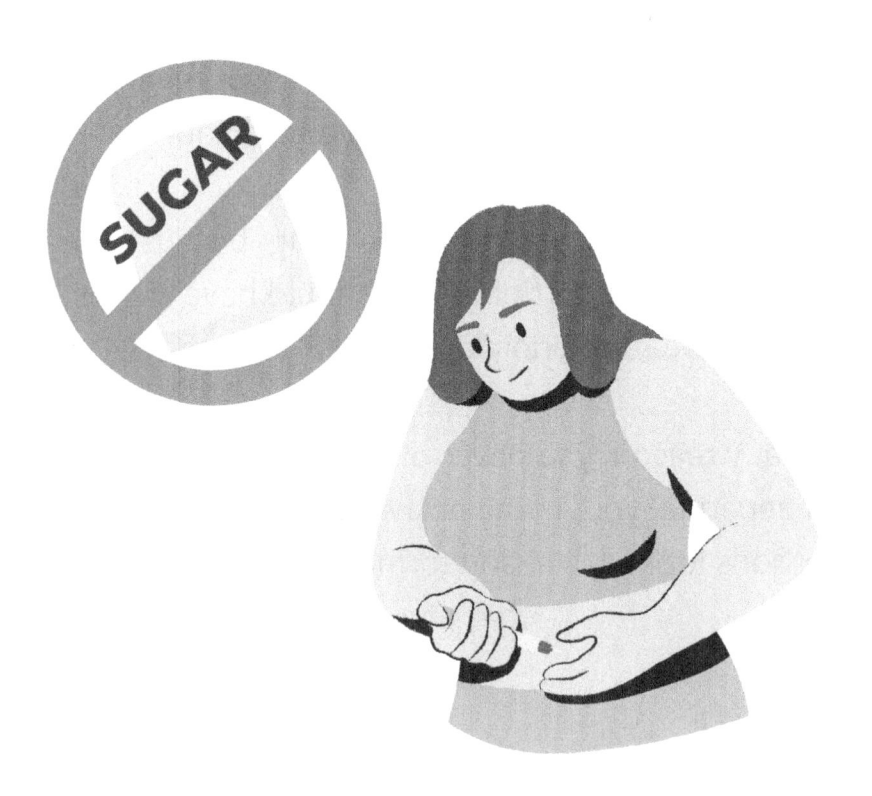

Chapter Eight
Why Sugar Is The Enemy of Health

For all my talk about Fiber being a "Good Carb"... I want to now talk about the most horrible carb. Sugar has earned a notorious reputation as the, "evil carb," and not just by me.

This chapter explains in detail how excessive sugar consumption is linked to a wide array of health problems.

Modern diets, particularly in Western societies, have seen a dramatic increase in added sugars, which in turn has been associated with metabolic disturbances, cognitive decline, oral health issues, and even increased cancer risks.

The body does not discriminate when it comes to processing sugar; the very same molecule that fuels our cells can, when overconsumed, set off a cascade of negative physiological reactions.

At the core of the issue is the way sugar affects our metabolism. Consuming sugar causes rapid, roller-coaster spikes in blood glucose levels, which leads to surges in insulin secretion.

Over time, the body becomes less responsive to insulin — a condition known as insulin resistance — which is a precursor to type 2 diabetes and contributes to obesity.

This metabolic imbalance creates an environment in which chronic low-grade inflammation becomes more common, setting the stage for various chronic diseases.

Numerous studies have demonstrated that sustained high levels of sugar in the diet can disrupt normal metabolic processes, thereby increasing the likelihood of developing metabolic syndrome and cardiovascular disease.

The effects of sugar extend well beyond the realm of metabolic health. Emerging evidence suggests that high sugar intake can also have detrimental effects on the brain. Elevated blood sugar levels and insulin resistance are linked to an increased risk of cognitive decline and dementia.

Research has indicated that excess sugar may accelerate the formation of advanced glycation end products (**AGEs**), which can cause oxidative stress and inflammation in brain tissue, thereby impairing cognitive functions.

These findings are part of a growing body of literature that implicates diet as a modifiable risk factor for dementia and other neurodegenerative disorders.

Oral health is another area where sugar exerts its destructive influence. When sugar is consumed, bacteria in the mouth metabolize it and produce acids as a byproduct. These acids erode tooth enamel, leading to cavities, tooth decay, and gum disease.

The presence of sugar in the oral environment not only supports the growth of harmful bacteria but can also result in persistent bad breath and an overall decline in dental health.

The link between dietary sugars and poor oral hygiene is well-documented in dental research and remains a significant concern for public health.

Beyond metabolic, cognitive, and dental effects, sugar is a key contributor to chronic inflammation.

Inflammation is the body's natural response to injury or infection, but when it becomes chronic, it is implicated in a host of diseases.

High levels of circulating sugar have been shown to increase inflammatory markers, such as C-reactive protein, which further stress bodily systems and can exacerbate existing health problems.

Inflammation is a common underlying mechanism that **links sugar consumption to a range of illnesses**, reinforcing the idea that reducing sugar intake may alleviate many of these inflammatory conditions.

Moreover, it's important to recognize the a few specific examples of "illnesses" I am referring to, when saying they are linked to sugar consumption.

Type 2 diabetes is a major metabolic disorder that arises from chronic high blood sugar levels and insulin resistance, and it is frequently accompanied by obesity. That linked illness is so obvious & well-documented, that Im sure most of you already knew that.

However, some lesser obvious illnesses would include, but are not limited to...

Non-alcoholic fatty liver disease, characterized by the build-up of fat in liver cells, is another condition strongly associated with high sugar intake, particularly from fructose, and can progress to serious liver inflammation and scarring.

Additionally, cardiovascular conditions such as coronary artery disease and hypertension have been linked to diets rich in added sugars.

There's also growing evidence that excessive sugar intake contributes to neurodegenerative diseases like Alzheimer's, and may increase the risk of certain cancers, including breast, colon, and pancreatic cancer, by creating a pro-inflammatory environment that fosters tumor growth.

The association between sugar and cancer is often oversimplified by the statement that, "cancer cells love sugar."

While it is true that all cells, including malignant ones, require glucose for energy, the relationship between sugar consumption and cancer is complex.

Elevated blood sugar and insulin levels can lead to increased production of insulin-like growth factors, which may promote tumor growth.

Furthermore, a high-sugar diet contributes to obesity, a well-established risk factor for several types of cancer.

Although sugar does not directly cause cancer, **its role in fostering an environment that supports cancer cell proliferation and growth** is a significant concern in the medical community.

Adding to these multifaceted concerns is the **addictive nature** of sugar.
Consumption of sugar triggers the brain's reward system, leading to the release of dopamine — a neurotransmitter associated with pleasure and satisfaction.

This immediate gratification reinforces the desire for further sugar intake, establishing a cycle that mirrors other forms of addiction.

Specifically, repeated exposure to sugar can lead to alterations in the brain regions involved in reward and decision-making, such as the nucleus accumbens and prefrontal cortex.

These changes create a dependency where the brain craves the quick energy boost and emotional lift that sugar provides, making it exceedingly difficult for individuals to reduce or eliminate sugar from their diets.

The rapid energy surges followed by inevitable crashes only serve to perpetuate this cycle, as the body seeks to regain that fleeting sense of well-being.

Such neurological and physiological responses explain why many struggle to give up sugar, despite being aware of its harmful impacts.

However, as we discussed in chapter three, the way GLP-1 injections impact **Neurotransmitter Interactions**, and helps us fight addictions as a result of that, being on these medications can make it easier to give up sugar. That alone would have a significant positive impact on your health & prevent further future health issues.

In conclusion, the evidence linking excessive sugar consumption, or even just normal consumption on a regular basis over time, to a wide spectrum of health problems is robust and multifaceted.

From its role in metabolic dysfunction and cognitive decline to its contribution to poor oral health, chronic inflammation, and the promotion of a pro-cancer environment, sugar presents a formidable challenge to public health.

Plus, the addictive properties of sugar further complicate efforts to reduce intake, trapping individuals in a cycle that not only affects physical health but also impacts overall quality of life.

A conscious effort to reduce added sugars can lead to significant improvements in overall well-being and a reduced risk of many of the ailments that plague modern society.

This underscores the critical importance of dietary choices, and provides a compelling case for rethinking our relationship with sugar, in pursuit of better long-term health outcomes.

Chapter Nine
Weightlifting & Resistance Training

Weightlifting and resistance training are foundational elements in a comprehensive weight loss and health improvement strategy.

While GLP-1 medications and a balanced diet offer powerful tools by reducing appetite and stabilizing blood sugar levels, exercise — particularly structured strength training — plays a critical role in preserving muscle mass, enhancing metabolism, and sculpting a strong, toned physique.

Integrating resistance training into your routine not only supports weight loss by ensuring that fat, rather than precious muscle tissue, is shed, but it also contributes to overall health by fostering strength, endurance, and a more resilient body.

During periods of calorie restriction, the body is prone to losing muscle along with fat, a phenomenon that can compromise metabolic health and overall strength.

Resistance training combats this issue by stimulating muscle protein synthesis, the process by which the body repairs and builds new muscle fibers.

This regenerative activity ensures that the loss in body weight is predominantly from fat stores rather than lean muscle tissue.

In fact, consistent engagement in weightlifting can result in actual gains in lean muscle mass, which not only enhances physical strength but also contributes to a more efficient metabolism.

Muscle tissue is metabolically active, meaning it burns more calories at rest compared to fat tissue, thereby increasing the basal metabolic rate.

An elevated metabolism is essential for maintaining weight loss, as it allows the body to better manage energy fluctuations and adapt to changes in dietary intake.

In addition to preserving muscle mass, resistance training offers a host of benefits that extend well beyond the scale.

By building strength, individuals gain the capacity to perform daily activities with greater ease and reduced risk of injury. Enhanced muscular strength also supports joint health and overall mobility, making everyday tasks less taxing and improving quality of life.

The process of lifting weights imposes a healthy stress on the muscles, encouraging them to adapt and become more resilient. This adaptation not only translates to improved physical performance but also contributes to the maintenance of a toned and balanced physique over the long term.

A well-structured resistance training routine should be viewed as an integral component of a sustainable weight loss program. Consistency is key; engaging in strength training sessions at least two to three times per week allows the body to recover adequately while continuously challenging the muscles.

Incorporating a variety of exercises that target major muscle groups — from compound movements like squats, deadlifts, and bench presses to isolation exercises that focus on smaller muscle groups — ensures balanced development and prevents the onset of plateaus.

This variety also keeps the training regimen dynamic and engaging, which can be crucial for long-term adherence.

When the body is exposed to diverse movement patterns and resistance levels, it adapts by becoming stronger and more efficient, paving the way for improved performance in both daily activities and specialized workouts.

The synergistic effects of combining resistance training with GLP-1 medications and proper nutrition cannot be overstated.

While GLP-1 medications work by suppressing appetite and aiding in blood sugar regulation, they do not distinguish between fat and muscle when it comes to weight loss. Resistance training acts as a safeguard, ensuring that the weight lost through dietary changes and medication is predominantly fat rather than muscle.

When this exercise is paired with a high-protein diet, it supports optimal muscle repair and growth. Proteins provide the essential building blocks needed for the synthesis of new muscle fibers, thereby enhancing recovery after strenuous workouts.

This integrated approach results in a **powerful cycle of improvement:** the medication and diet facilitate weight loss, resistance training preserves and builds muscle, and enhanced muscle mass in turn elevates metabolic rate, creating a sustainable environment for long-term health and fitness.

Resistance training also plays a pivotal role in establishing sustainable energy levels.

A robust metabolic rate, fostered by increased muscle mass, means that the body can efficiently convert food into energy, even at rest.

Let me clarify that for a moment! If you gain muscle mass, the fuel (energy) it requires to maintain that muscle mass — means that you could still be burning calories & fat, even when you're sitting at the computer or sleeping at night. "At Rest"... Muscle mass naturally helps prevent fat (weight regain) by burning through it.

This improved energy efficiency allows individuals to better handle fluctuations in their daily routines, from unexpected challenges to variations in dietary intake.

Over time, the cumulative benefits of regular weightlifting extend to improved cardiovascular health, reduced risk of chronic diseases, and enhanced mental well-being.

The psychological boost that comes from increased strength and physical capability can be as significant as the physiological benefits, contributing to a more confident and resilient mindset.

Ultimately, weightlifting and resistance training are not mere adjuncts to a weight loss program; they are indispensable components that ensure the quality of the weight lost is optimal for overall health.

They offer a multi-dimensional approach to weight management by preserving lean muscle, elevating metabolic function, and fostering a strong and agile body.

When combined with the appetite-suppressing benefits of GLP-1 medications and a balanced, protein-rich diet, resistance training forms the cornerstone of a long-term strategy for health, fitness, and well-being.

This integrated methodology not only supports the immediate goal of weight loss but also lays the groundwork for a lifetime of improved physical performance and vitality.

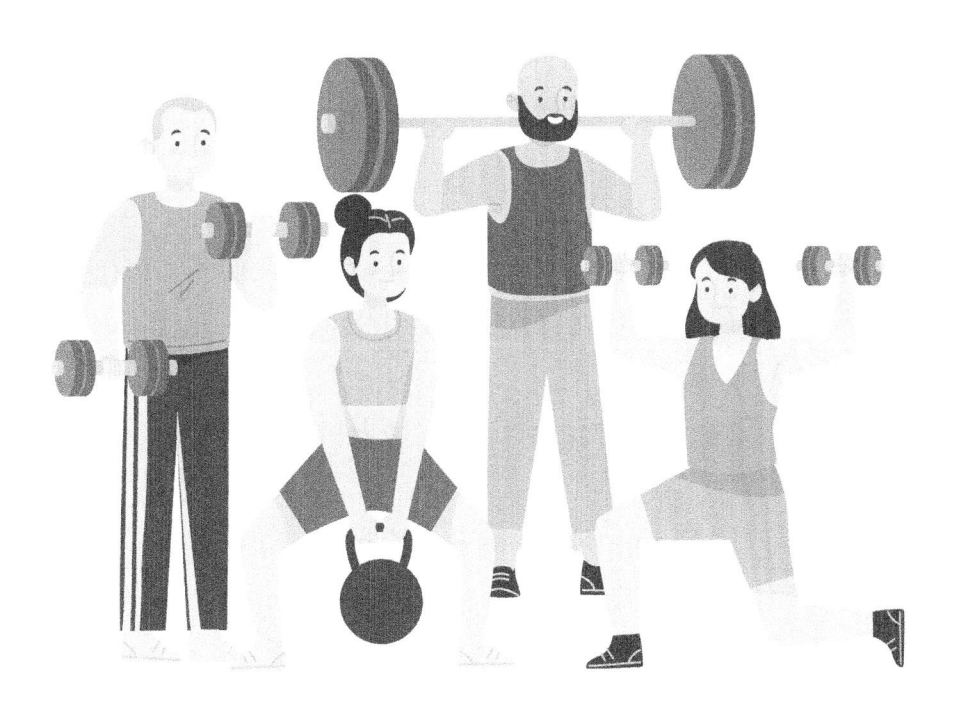

Chapter Ten
Building Strength

Muscle retention is a critical aspect of sustainable weight loss.

In this chapter, we delve into the science behind muscle preservation and how resistance training works in tandem with nutritional strategies — particularly a high-protein diet — to maintain and even build lean muscle during weight loss.

Understanding this science not only empowers you to optimize your training but also reinforces the importance of muscle for metabolic health.

The Science of Muscle Retention

1. Muscle Protein Synthesis (MPS)

What It Is: Muscle protein synthesis is the process by which the body repairs and builds muscle fibers after exercise.

Stimulating MPS: Resistance training acts as a powerful stimulus for MPS, which is further enhanced by adequate protein intake.

2. The Role of Satellite Cells

Muscle Regeneration: Satellite cells, which are dormant cells located on muscle fibers, become activated during exercise. They play a crucial role in repairing damaged muscle and contributing to muscle growth.

Enhanced Adaptation: Regular weightlifting increases the number and activity of satellite cells, promoting muscle regeneration and strengthening.

3. Hormonal Influence

Anabolic Hormones: Resistance training boosts the production of anabolic hormones like testosterone and growth hormone, which are essential for muscle growth and repair.

Synergy with Diet: A diet rich in protein provides the necessary amino acids for these hormones to work effectively, ensuring optimal muscle retention.

Optimizing Your Training and Nutrition

1. Integrating Strength Workouts

Structured Programs: Develop a structured resistance training program that gradually increases in intensity.

This progressive overload is key to continually challenging your muscles.

Balanced Routine: Incorporate both compound movements (e.g., squats, deadlifts) and isolation exercises to target specific muscles.

2. Nutritional Support for Muscle Growth

Protein Timing: Consume a protein-rich meal or shake within 30-60 minutes after your workout to maximize muscle repair.

Consistent Intake: Spread your protein intake throughout the day to maintain a steady supply of amino acids, supporting continuous muscle protein synthesis.

Building strength and preserving muscle are cornerstones of a sustainable weight loss plan.

By understanding the science behind muscle retention and combining targeted resistance training with a high protein diet, you can safeguard your lean muscle mass and enhance your overall metabolic rate.

This scientific foundation ensures that your weight loss journey not only results in a leaner physique but also in a stronger, more resilient body.

Cardio vs. Strength Training

Cardio versus strength training is like choosing between two superhero allies on your weight loss journey—each has its unique powers, and together they form an unstoppable team.

Imagine cardio as the energetic speedster, always ready to boost your heart health, increase endurance, and torch calories in the moment.

Whether you're jogging in the park, dancing in a Zumba class, or even cycling to work, cardiovascular exercise gets your heart pumping and your blood flowing, transforming every workout into a fat-burning fiesta.

When you engage in cardio, you're not just burning calories during the session; you're setting the stage for overall fat loss by increasing your daily energy expenditure.

This constant calorie burn, paired with smart dietary choices, can help reduce excess body fat, making cardio an essential component of any well-rounded fitness program.

By engaging in regular resistance training, you not only keep your muscles intact but also add new muscle, which boosts your resting metabolic rate.

This means that even when you're fast asleep, your body is quietly burning calories, setting the stage for long-term weight management and preventing the dreaded cycle of losing progress once dietary or medication strategies like GLP-1s change course.

Now, here's where the magic really happens: balancing these two forms of exercise. Think of it as mixing the right ingredients in a recipe to get the perfect outcome.

Too much cardio without strength training can lead to muscle loss, leaving you with a lean but flabby physique.

Conversely, focusing solely on weights might boost your muscle mass but won't give you that quick, heart-pumping burst that helps shed calories during the workout.

The sweet spot is in integrating **both** modalities into your routine...

For instance, you might dedicate two to three days a week to weightlifting sessions that target major muscle groups — squats, deadlifts, bench presses, and rows — while carving out another couple of days for cardiovascular activities that get your heart rate soaring.

This integrated approach not only maximizes calorie burn during your workouts but also ensures that the muscle you work so hard to build remains intact and even flourishes, safeguarding your metabolism for the long haul.

It's important to tailor your exercise strategy to your personal goals and schedule. If your primary aim is to boost cardiovascular health or prepare for a marathon, cardio might take a more central role in your workout plan.

However, even in that scenario, incorporating strength training is crucial to prevent muscle loss and maintain a balanced physique.

For those of us juggling busy schedules, combining cardio and strength training in one session might be the answer.

High-intensity interval training (HIIT) or circuit training, for example, allows you to reap the benefits of both worlds in a shorter amount of time.

These workouts blend bursts of cardiovascular activity with periods of resistance exercises, keeping your heart rate elevated while engaging multiple muscle groups simultaneously. It's a time-efficient and effective strategy that can transform even the busiest day into a productive fitness session.

When it comes to planning your workouts, consistency and recovery are key. Designing a weekly schedule that thoughtfully alternates between cardio and strength sessions can help you avoid overtraining and reduce the risk of injury.

Listen to your body — if you're feeling fatigued, it might be time for an active recovery day, a brisk walk, or some gentle stretching to keep the momentum going without pushing too hard. Monitoring your progress is another vital piece of the puzzle.

Keep track of your performance, whether that's through a fitness journal, a wearable device, or simply by noticing changes in how your clothes fit.

Over time, as your endurance improves and your muscles become more defined, you might find that your workout routine needs tweaking to keep up with your evolving fitness level.

This process of continuous adjustment is part of a holistic approach to health that values cardiovascular fitness, muscular strength, flexibility, and overall endurance.

In essence, understanding the distinct benefits of cardiovascular exercise and strength training allows you to design an exercise regimen that is both effective and enjoyable.

Cardio ignites your body's calorie-burning engine and strengthens your heart, while resistance training builds the muscular foundation that keeps your metabolism humming.

Together, these two forms of exercise complement each other perfectly, ensuring that you not only lose fat but also preserve—and even build—the lean muscle that supports long-term weight management.

Whether you're on GLP-1 medications or simply striving for a healthier lifestyle, balancing cardio with strength training is key to creating a resilient, toned, and energetic body.

Embrace the journey, have fun with your workouts, and remember that each step, sprint, and lift brings you closer to a healthier, happier you.

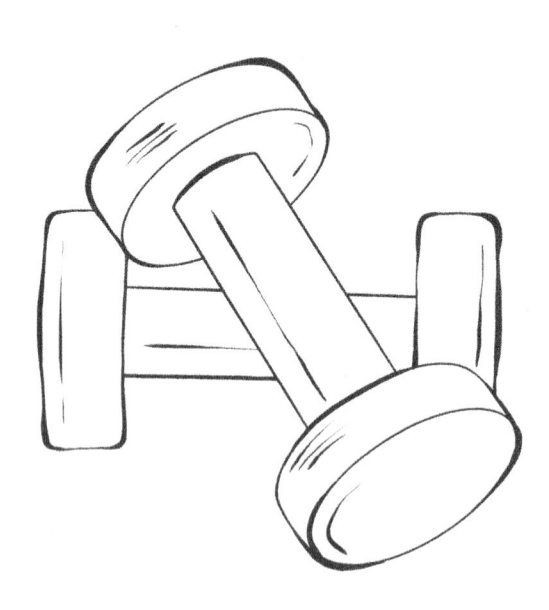

Chapter Eleven
Preventing Plateaus – Keeping Progress Steady

Preventing plateaus is a bit like finding yourself cruising on a scenic highway only to discover that you've hit a long, flat stretch where the scenery seems to stall—and so does your progress.

In the weight loss journey, this plateau can feel frustrating, almost as if your body has hit a stubborn speed bump.

But the truth is, plateaus are a natural part of any transformation process, a signal that your body is adapting, and with the right strategies, you can break through them and keep your momentum strong.

One of the primary culprits behind these stagnant periods is metabolic adaptation. As you shed pounds, your body naturally becomes more efficient at using energy, much like upgrading from a gas-guzzling car to one that sips fuel delicately.

This efficiency is rooted in survival instincts; your body adjusts to a lower calorie intake and reduced body mass by slowing down its metabolism. It's a bit like your engine learning to run on less, conserving energy for the long haul.

While this is a brilliant survival mechanism in evolutionary terms, it does make further weight loss a tougher challenge. When your metabolism gets into this energy-saving mode, the calories you once burned easily now seem to vanish less readily, which can lead to a plateau in your progress.

Exercise adaptation also plays a significant role. Over time, your body becomes a master of routine. The same exercises that once pushed you to break a sweat can start to feel like old friends who no longer surprise you.

This phenomenon, known as routine familiarity, means that the body gets accustomed to the stimulus and stops responding with the same vigor.

As the gains in strength and calorie burn begin to diminish, it might feel as if you're stuck in a loop, performing the same routine with diminishing results.

The solution lies in shaking things up...
challenging your muscles in new ways and forcing them to adapt once again. Just like adding a twist to your favorite dance move, varying your workouts can reawaken your body's potential for progress.

So, what can you do when you find your weight loss journey stalling?
The first step is to adjust your nutrition.
As your body weight decreases, so do your caloric needs. It's a good idea to periodically reassess your calorie intake to ensure it aligns with your new metabolic demands. Think of it as recalibrating your fuel gauge; what worked when you were heavier may now be slightly excessive.

Along with total calories, tweaking your macronutrient ratios can be a game-changer.

For instance, increasing your protein intake slightly can help support muscle maintenance and even boost your metabolic rate. Protein is like the unsung hero in your diet — it repairs and builds muscle, which in turn keeps your metabolism humming even when you're resting.

Modifying your exercise routine is another powerful strategy.

Progressive overload, the practice of gradually increasing the intensity or resistance in your workouts, is key to keeping your muscles on their toes.

By pushing your muscles a little harder than before, you force them to adapt, spurring continued strength gains and a higher metabolic rate.

Variation is also critical. Switching from steady-state cardio to high-intensity interval training (HIIT), for example, can provide a fresh burst of energy and stimulate your metabolism in new ways. And don't underestimate the value of rest and recovery.

Sometimes, a plateau isn't a sign of failure but a quiet call from your body for more recovery time. Integrating active recovery days, where you engage in lighter activities like walking or yoga, can prevent overtraining and set the stage for your next breakthrough.

Tracking your progress with a keen eye is another essential piece of the puzzle.

Keeping detailed records of your workouts, body measurements, and dietary intake can offer you invaluable insights.

It's like being your own detective — analyzing the clues to identify what might be holding you back and where small adjustments can yield big results.

Over time, as you notice patterns and shifts in your body composition, you'll be better equipped to tweak your routine and nutrition, ensuring that every aspect of your approach evolves with your progress.

Equally important is cultivating the right mindset. It's easy to get discouraged when the scale seems stuck, but remember, plateaus are a natural part of any weight loss journey.

They're not a reflection of your commitment or potential — they're simply a sign that your body is adapting.

Embrace these moments with a positive, patient attitude, knowing that strategic adjustments will eventually lead to renewed progress.

Think of your journey like a video game where each level presents new challenges; with every plateau, you're simply leveling up your understanding of what your body needs to succeed.

In the grand scheme, preventing plateaus isn't about constantly battling against your body—it's about working with it.

Stay flexible in your approach, and don't be afraid to experiment with different workout intensities, nutritional tweaks, or even rest patterns.

Your weight loss journey is dynamic, and so should be your strategies. By embracing the need for periodic changes and viewing plateaus as opportunities to fine-tune your routine, you can maintain steady progress and keep your transformation on track.

Ultimately, the key to preventing plateaus and keeping progress steady lies in understanding your body's signals and adapting your approach accordingly.

By adjusting your nutrition, varying your exercise routines, and monitoring your progress with a positive mindset, you create a sustainable framework for long-term success.

So, when you hit that inevitable flat stretch, remember that it's not a setback but a stepping stone — an invitation to reexamine, recalibrate, and emerge even stronger on your journey to a healthier, leaner you.

Enjoy the process, have fun with the experiments, and keep moving forward, one smart adjustment at a time.

If your plateau persist after you have continued to workout and eat correctly... If you have tried to switch things up, but are still not having luck... And maybe you're noticing a little increase in your appetite coming back?

THIS IS WHEN YOU FINALLY DECIDE TO TITRATE UP IN DOSAGE!

Increasing your dose should be a last resort, while you are still on your journey with more weight to lose! Take your time going up in dosage.

Chapter Twelve
Beyond the Scale: Measuring True Success

Embarking on a weight loss journey often means fixating on the numbers the scale displays.

That number can feel like a badge of honor or a source of constant anxiety, but focusing solely on weight is like reading just one chapter of a very rich novel — it hardly tells the whole story.

True, sustainable success encompasses so much more than a single, fluctuating number. It involves understanding body composition, recognizing increased energy levels, celebrating strength gains, and appreciating overall well-being.

In this chapter, we'll explore why the scale can be misleading, how to track real progress, and why shifting your focus can lead to a healthier, more resilient mindset.

It's undeniable that watching the scale dip can be incredibly satisfying.

However, if you're only looking at that one measurement, you might miss the myriad of changes happening within your body.

Daily weight fluctuations are completely normal — one day you might be up a pound or two even if you haven't changed a thing.

These variations can be due to water retention, hormonal shifts (especially for those with monthly cycles), or even something as mundane as the weight of the food and liquids in your system.

Trust me when I say, sometimes you might just need to drop off a pound's worth of... well, you know! (Poop)

That's why many of us opt to weigh ourselves first thing in the morning, butt-ass naked after our first pee, to get the most accurate reading, before any external factors come into play.

It's important to understand that if the number stays the same or even goes up slightly, it's perfectly okay. The scale is only one snapshot in a much larger picture.

When we hone in solely on the scale, we risk falling into the trap of unrealistic expectations. The singular focus on weight can lead to frustration and disappointment, even if other key health indicators are showing remarkable improvement.

For instance, as you lose fat and build muscle through exercise and proper nutrition, you might not see a dramatic drop in your weight because muscle is denser than fat.

This means you could be looking leaner and feeling stronger, yet the scale might not reflect that transformation.

It's like judging a book solely by its cover; the true narrative of your progress is written in how you feel, how your clothes fit, and how much more energy you have day to day.

One of the most valuable ways to gauge progress is by emphasizing body composition over sheer weight. Body composition, which considers the ratio of fat to lean muscle, provides a much clearer picture of your overall fitness.

A decrease in body fat percentage — even if the scale remains stubbornly steady — is a powerful indicator of improved health.

Various methods, such as bioelectrical impedance analysis, DEXA scans, or even simple skinfold measurements, can help you track these changes over time.

As you continue to exercise, particularly through strength training, you're not just losing weight; you're reshaping your body.

Lean muscle not only enhances your physical appearance by creating a more toned and defined look, but it also ramps up your metabolism.

Muscle tissue burns calories at rest, meaning that your body is working around the clock to keep you fit — even while you sleep!

Also bare in mind, muscle can weigh more than fat on the scale. So it can be you losing weight, the numbers go down overall, but every so often the number goes up again.

Not because you're regaining fat, but getting leaner & gaining muscle. That's a good thing!

Beyond these physical metrics, it's essential to celebrate non-scale victories (**NSVs**) — those meaningful, everyday improvements that the scale simply can't capture.

NSVs include things like improved endurance during your workouts, better quality sleep, clearer mental focus, or simply feeling more confident in your own skin.

Maybe you've discovered that you can run a little longer, lift a little heavier, or that your clothes are fitting in a way they never did before. These victories are the real trophies of your journey.

They are moments that remind you of how far you've come and serve as powerful motivators to keep pushing forward. Start journaling your progress — note those small wins and milestones.

Write down how you feel after a workout, how your energy levels have improved, or even the compliments you receive on your glowing skin and healthy hair.

These reflections not only document your journey but also help reinforce the positive changes happening in your life.

Adopting a holistic approach to measuring success means integrating multiple metrics into your evaluation process. Instead of relying solely on the scale, combine it with body composition assessments, NSVs, and other health markers such as blood pressure, cholesterol levels, and blood sugar control.

Taking a before photo can be particularly illuminating — sometimes, a visual reminder is all it takes to see the tremendous progress you've made, even if the scale hasn't budged as much as you'd like.

Regularly reviewing these varied data points offers a comprehensive perspective on your transformation. It underscores that your journey isn't just about losing pounds; it's about gaining health, vitality, and a renewed zest for life.

Perhaps most importantly, shifting your mindset is key to embracing true success. Real progress is measured over the long term, not by a quick fix or a number on a scale.

Sustainable changes in body composition, increased strength, and enhanced overall well-being are the real victories that lead to lasting transformation. Understand that progress can be slow, non-linear, and sometimes even frustrating — but every step forward, no matter how small, is a win.

Resilience and adaptation are the hallmarks of any worthwhile journey, and by focusing on multiple markers of success, you'll find it easier to stay motivated and inspired.

In the end, your weight loss journey is about so much more than what the scale tells you. It's about celebrating the improvements in your physical fitness, the energy that lights up your day, and the growing strength that makes every challenge a little easier.

By looking beyond the scale and valuing the comprehensive benefits of your lifestyle changes, you cultivate a more positive mindset and a healthier relationship with your body.

Every muscle gained, every extra minute of energy, and every moment of feeling truly well is a testament to your dedication and hard work. So, keep your eyes on the broader picture and remember that every victory — scale or non-scale — is a step toward a healthier, happier, and more vibrant you.

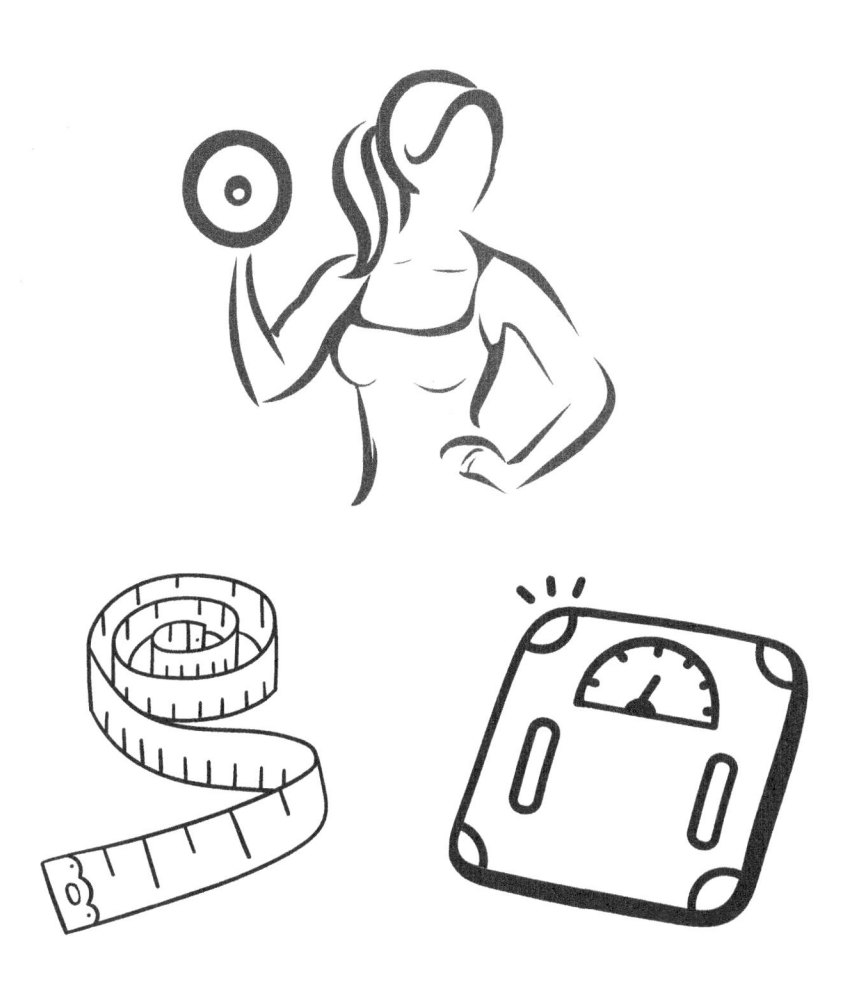

Chapter Thirteen
Mindset Matters: The Psychology of Long-Term Weight Loss

Embarking on a weight loss journey is a bit like setting out on an epic road trip — you've got your map, your fuel (hello, diet and exercise), and even a few fancy gadgets like GLP-1 medications to help you along the way.

But if you've ever taken a long drive, you know that the journey isn't just about the destination; it's also about the mindset you bring along for the ride.

In this chapter, we're diving headfirst into the psychology of long-term weight loss, because while your body can change, your mindset is the engine that drives sustainable transformation.

So buckle up, grab your favorite healthy snack, and get ready to learn why your thoughts are just as important as your workout routine.

The first hurdle on our journey is overcoming mental barriers. Imagine your mind as a bustling city where some of the residents — those pesky negative thoughts — can really slow down progress.

Many of us have experienced that inner dialogue that whispers, "I can't change" or "I'll always be overweight."

Recognizing these limiting beliefs is like catching a speed camera on your road trip — you might get a little startled at first, but it's a crucial wake-up call to adjust your course.

Instead of letting these negative thoughts dictate your journey, try reframing your narrative.

Replace "I always fail" with "Every setback is a lesson in disguise." Yes, even that time you overindulged on a tub of ice cream (Hey, I've been there & done that! Coffee Flavored Ice Cream was my weakness back then.) can be seen as a learning opportunity, rather than a catastrophic failure.

Humor, after all, is a powerful antidote to self-doubt.

Another significant mental barrier is emotional eating, which, let's be honest, many of us have a love-hate relationship with.

When life throws curveballs — be it stress, boredom, or anxiety — turning to food for comfort can seem like the easiest escape.

But here's a truth bomb: using food to cope with emotions rarely leads to lasting comfort. If your history includes moments where food was your go-to for managing tough times, know that you're not alone.

And if past trauma has contributed to unhealthy eating habits, please consider seeking help from a professional.

Therapy isn't a sign of weakness — it's a way to build stronger emotional muscles.

Meanwhile, try keeping a food and mood diary. It might sound a bit "out there," but writing down what you eat alongside how you feel can help you identify patterns. Journaling is a WONDERFUL idea, and strong tool to use on your journey.

Once you see the triggers, you can develop alternative strategies: take a brisk walk, practice mindfulness, or dive into a hobby that makes you feel alive.

Trust me, replacing that emotional rollercoaster with a burst of endorphins from a fun activity is a game changer.

Now, let's talk about building a positive and resilient mindset. It's easy to get caught up in grand visions of instant success, but long-term weight loss is more like tending to a garden than sprinting a marathon.

Setting realistic goals is key. Instead of dreaming about losing 50 pounds overnight (unless you're in a superhero movie), focus on short-term objectives that are attainable and measurable.

Celebrate each small victory — whether it's choosing a healthy snack over a bag of chips or finally nailing that yoga pose you've been practicing for weeks.

When you focus on the process rather than just the outcome, every step forward feels like progress, and your confidence grows with each healthy habit you cement.

Self-compassion is your best friend on this journey. Embrace the fact that you're human — setbacks are normal and perfectly okay. There will be days when you feel like you've taken one step forward and two steps back, and that's fine.

Think of it as a quirky dance; sometimes you stumble, but you get back up and keep grooving.

Positive reinforcement can go a long way: celebrate your successes, both big and small. Whether it's a compliment from a friend or simply the fact that you felt more energetic during your workout, every bit of progress deserves recognition.

And while it's tempting to reward yourself with a slice of cake after a hard day, try to choose non-food rewards that nurture your overall well-being — a new workout outfit, a spa day, or even just a few quiet moments with your favorite book.

Of course, no journey is complete without a strong support system. Building a network of people who understand and encourage your efforts is like having your own personal pit crew.

And remember, while doctors are supposed to be medical professionals, we like to view them as experts. However, they're human just like you & me! They can be wrong, or have opinions about certain medications & health choices, too!

If one opinion doesn't quite resonate with you, or you feel like they aren't educated on a matter the way they should be... Maybe you dont feel supported by this doctor enough to open up to them & create a safe & effective plan... Then don't hesitate to get a second opinion. Try another doctor if possible, until you find one that feels right for you!

Find those who get it, who know about GLP-1 medications and the challenges of weight loss, and who offer advice without judgment.

Additionally, joining communities — whether online or in-person — can provide a treasure trove of shared experiences, tips, and much-needed pep talks when you're feeling down.

After all, it's easier to face the uphill battles when you know others are on the same trail with you.

Finally, let's embrace the power of a growth mindset. In the world of weight loss, setbacks aren't the end of the story; they're just plot twists that make the narrative more interesting.

Each challenge is an opportunity to learn, refine your strategies, and come back stronger. Maintain an openness to new ideas — whether it's a novel workout routine, a fresh dietary approach, or simply a new way to think about food — and be willing to adapt as you discover what works best for you.

Continuous improvement is not about perfection; it's about progress. So, when you stumble, laugh it off, learn from it, and keep moving forward. Remember, every great story has its ups and downs, and your journey is no exception.

In conclusion, the mental aspect of weight loss is just as crucial as the physical components.

By overcoming limiting beliefs, managing emotional eating, setting realistic goals, and building a supportive network, you lay a solid psychological foundation for long-term success.

Your mindset isn't merely a tool for tackling obstacles — it's the driving force behind every healthy decision you make.

Embrace it, nurture it, and let it propel you toward a healthier, happier future. With the right attitude and a sprinkle of humor along the way, you'll find that sustainable weight loss is not only achievable — it's also an adventure worth savoring.

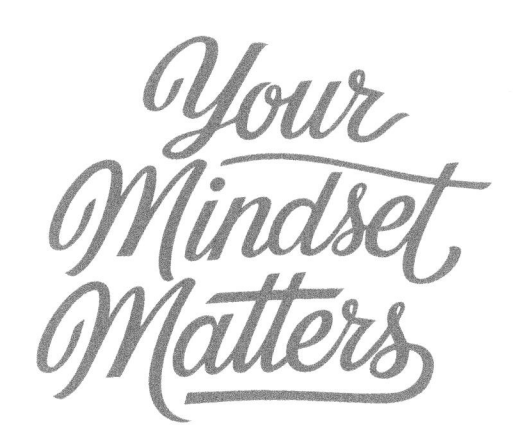

Your Mindset Matters

Chapter Fourteen
The Truth About "Semaglutide Face & Butt"

I'm gonna level with you, I have compassion for those of us who are on our journeys. I do not have compassion for intentional ignorance; by people trying to drag us down via spreading the myths, exaggerated risks for the sake of fear mongering, & misinformation!

I will try to remain tactful in this chapter, but Im going to be unapologically blunt.

Let me start by saying, "Haters gonna hate!"

There are plenty of people out there parroting the same tired, uninformed nonsense about GLP-1 injections as if they're the ultimate authority on weight loss.

Newsflash: most of these wannabe "experts" running their mouths (especially online) haven't even dipped their toes into the GLP-1 pool. They've never used it, and never did any legitimate research on it.

The terms "Semaglutide Face" and "Semaglutide Butt" have been thrown around by those who either don't understand, or are too envious of the progress folks are making with GLP-1 medications.

These labels are nothing more than misnomers, **born out of resentment** from people who'd rather see you fail than celebrate your victories.

And are then **spread further** by those who failed to go educate themselves on the topic, and wanted to join the bandwagon of haters to feel like they're part of something.

And honestly, guess what? Not everyone wants to see you succeed. This is a sad & cold reality people losing weight endure at some point. Because it can unfortunately include friends & family sometimes.

It'll suck. It'll sting. But you have to ignore the noise and focus on your journey. Let me repeat that!

NOT EVERYONE WANTS TO SEE YOU SUCCEED!
So just "do you," and forget those jerks. They're not worth your energy.
Do not let them derail you or discourage you!

Now, let's dive into the heart of the matter.

For starters, these labels weren't conjured up in a vacuum. They emerged from the murky depths of social media and anecdotal chatter, where unfounded claims spread faster than a viral meme.

People have taken a cursory glance at the dramatic changes that can accompany rapid weight loss and decided to blame the medication.

In reality, the supposed "Semaglutide Face" and "Semaglutide Butt" are simply the unintended side effects of shedding pounds at a breakneck pace — not the fault of the GLP-1 injections themselves.

Here's the truth: if you're losing weight quickly, your body isn't always given enough time to catch up. It's like trying to repackage a big ole blanket that was in vacuumed air-tight packaging — sometimes, things just don't go back!

Once that packaging was cut opened, and the blanket was able to fluff up with air, that was it!

The same goes for your skin. When you lose a significant amount of weight rapidly, your skin may struggle to retract smoothly all the way back down to it's original state.

This can result in loose or excess skin, particularly in areas like the face, abdomen, or even the butt.

But let's be real: isn't it better to have a bit of loose skin than to be trapped in the health issues that come with obesity?

The Role of Rapid Weight Loss

Rapid weight loss is a double-edged sword. On one side, it signals remarkable progress in reducing fat and improving metabolic health.

On the other, it can lead to excess skin formation because your body simply doesn't have the luxury of time to adjust.

Factors such as your age, genetics, and the total amount of weight lost all influence how your skin responds.

Younger skin with a robust supply of collagen and elastin tends to snap back better than skin that's been through decades of wear and tear.

So, while the medication is doing its job by curbing appetite and ramping up fat loss, the visible changes in your appearance are more about the speed of your transformation than any direct effect of the GLP-1 itself.

What the Science Says

Let's get down to the nuts and bolts of skin science. Your skin's elasticity depends on collagen and elastin — two proteins that give it structure and flexibility.

When you lose weight gradually, your skin has time to regenerate these proteins and adjust to your new shape.

Now, let's be crystal clear: GLP-1 medications like semaglutide work by regulating your appetite and metabolism. They're not magically remodeling your skin.

Any appearance changes are simply a byproduct of rapid weight loss. If your skin isn't retracting as fast as you'd like, it's not because the medication is altering your facial or body structure — it's because your body is adapting to a new reality.

In essence, GLP-1 is helping you win the battle against excess weight, and that, my friend, is a victory worth celebrating.

Practical Approaches to Managing Excess Skin

So, what can you do if you're worried about excess skin during your weight loss journey?

Incorporate Resistance Training: Strength training isn't just for bulking up — it helps preserve muscle mass and can improve your overall body composition. More muscle means a firmer, more sculpted appearance, which can mask the effects of loose skin. That skin used to be filled with fat. Now you can "fill it" with some toned muscle.

Nutritional Support for Skin Health: Don't forget about the vitamins and nutrients that keep your skin resilient.

Load up on foods rich in vitamin C, vitamin E, and collagen-boosting nutrients. Your skin will thank you for it. Also Stay hydrated! Studies show drinking lots of water improves the appearance of your skin.

Explore Skin-Firming Treatments: There are a variety of non-invasive treatments and skincare routines designed to boost skin elasticity. Whether it's firming creams, radiofrequency treatments, roller massage devices, or even just a dedicated skincare regimen... these options can help you feel more confident about your appearance, while helping your skin.

Moisturizing the body is important! Make it part of your nightly routine to apply skin-firming lotion to your arms, stomach, legs, and so on.

Set Realistic Expectations: Understand that some degree of loose skin may be an unavoidable part of significant weight loss.

Focus on the monumental health improvements you're making, rather than obsessing over perfection. At the end of the day, being healthy and happy trumps having a "perfect" physique.

Consult Professionals if Needed: If loose skin is a major concern, consider consulting with dermatologists or plastic surgeons who can offer personalized advice and treatment options.

Their guidance can be invaluable in managing your expectations and exploring corrective measures.

If you have 80 pounds or more to lose, chances are, you will have loose skin. These methods can help reduce the amount you have. The various methods can make it look better than it would have, had you done nothing to prevent excess skin.

However, you need to understand, significant weight loss will almost always result in needing to consult with a plastic surgeon afterwards, if you plan to get rid of it! Or you can choose to live with it, and not have it surgically removed. That is a personal choice.

I know that at some point, I would like to have a tummy tuck, because between four ginormous pregnancies followed by large weight loss, has resulted in my stomach having stretched out skin & a stretched out abdominal wall.

A "Perma-Pooch" is what I call it, and I want it gone, so I can finally see & enjoy the body I worked hard for.
To be able to see my real results, without my belly making me look much bigger than I should be for my weight. (Mainly due to the damaged abdominal wall hanging forward)

We only get to live this life once. I want to live it, feeling happy & confident in my own skin.
As we all do! If a tummy tuck with help make that happen for me, personally, I'm willing!

Others might not be willing, and that is okay too! Just make sure your choice is one that will bring **YOU** peace of mind, at the end of your health journey!

So to briefly recap:

The labels "Semaglutide Face" and "Semaglutide Butt" are nothing more than baseless buzzwords invented by people who would rather tear you down than lift you up. They represent the misguided attempts of those who fail to see the bigger picture — the transformation of your overall health.

At the end of the day, the journey of weight loss and better health is not about vanity — it's about living. Remaining alive, in a way that's healthier, and allows you to do things that the bigger obese you could not do or struggled with.

It's about reclaiming your health, your confidence, and your future. So if some extra skin is part of that price? Then so be it. You are gaining years of life, and that is worth everything.

Screw the haters, embrace the journey, and keep your eyes on what truly matters — your health, your happiness, and your future.

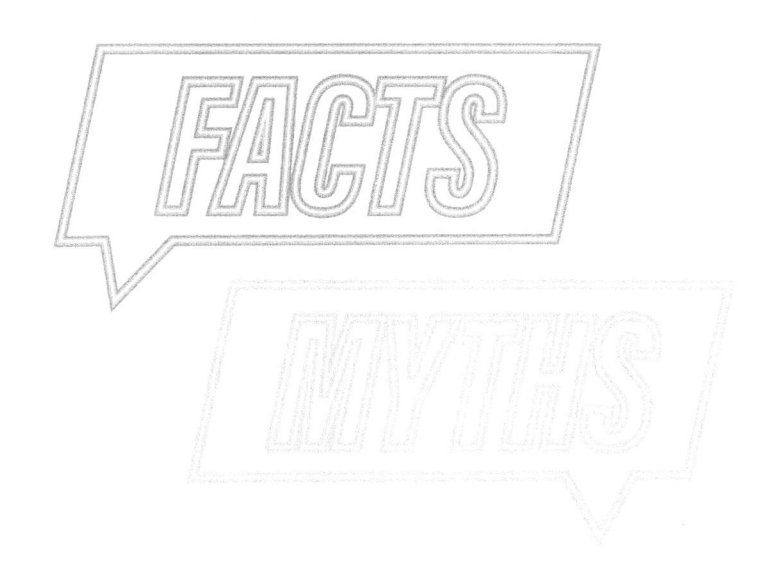

Chapter Fifteen
Debunking Myths & Addressing Controversies

In the world of health and wellness, few topics spark as much heated debate as weight loss medications.

Among them, GLP-1 therapies have earned a spotlight, both for their promising benefits and the persistent misconceptions that swirl around them.

In this chapter, we're going to roll up our sleeves, dive into the science, and debunk some of the most common myths — with a sprinkle of fun along the way.

Myth #1: GLP-1 Medications Are Just a "Starvation Diet"

One of the loudest myths in the arena is that being on a GLP-1 medication is akin to subjecting your body to a perpetual starvation mode.

Critics argue that rapid weight loss with these drugs is nothing more than muscle waste masquerading as fat loss. But let's clear the air.

That idea is a total misconception!

How They Really Work

GLP-1 medications work by enhancing your sense of satiety — that natural feeling of fullness that tells you, "Hey, you've had enough!" Rather than forcing your body into a state of nutritional deprivation, these drugs help you naturally lower your calorie intake.

You don't need quadruple the normal portion sizes, and 50 times the normal daily calorie intake, to be be considered well-fed! Eating until you feel full, is eating correctly. Not starving.

Here's the science in a nutshell:

Enhanced Satiety: By signaling to your brain that you're full, these medications reduce the urge to overeat.

Balanced Calorie Reduction: The reduction in food intake isn't about cutting calories down to a dangerously low level; it's about eating in a more mindful, sustainable way.

Preservation of Lean Muscle: Research shows that when GLP-1 therapy is combined with a high-protein diet and regular resistance training, the weight loss experienced is primarily from fat mass. Your muscles stay strong and intact, ready to support your active lifestyle.

So, instead of a "starvation diet," think of GLP-1 treatments as a tool that recalibrates your body's natural hunger signals — leading to healthier, more sustainable weight loss.

Myth #2: It's All About Eating 500 Calories a Day

Another frequent misconception is that users of GLP-1 medications are somehow surviving on a meager 500 calories per day, making the rapid weight loss seem unsustainable or unhealthy.
However, the reality is far more nuanced.

Beyond Calorie Counting
While reducing calorie intake is indeed a part of the equation, it's not the whole story.

The magic lies in how these medications help curb those pesky cravings that often derail even the best diet plans. They just aren't OVER EATING anymore.

When you're not fighting a constant battle with hunger, it's much easier to adopt a balanced eating pattern. On top of that, the temptation to reach for JUNK FOOD is greatly reduced. A person is not starving their self, just because they had the ability to ignore the cookies in the pantry.

Patients and research alike indicate that:
Appetite Suppression: The primary effect is a significant reduction in appetite, not a forced, ultra-low calorie regimen.

Sustainable Eating Habits: By reducing cravings, GLP-1 therapies support a more moderate and nutritionally balanced diet, helping you maintain energy levels and overall well-being.

It turns out that the success of GLP-1 medications isn't about extreme calorie restriction —

it's about empowering you to eat in a way that naturally leads to fat loss, without sacrificing the nutrients your body needs to thrive.

The Ethical Use Debate: Who Can Benefit?

Perhaps one of the most controversial discussions around GLP-1 medications is whether they should be reserved only for those who are overweight or have diabetes. Some argue that these drugs are a luxury only for a select few, but the emerging research paints a broader picture.

Expanding the Scope of Benefits

Recent studies and clinical practices have shown that the benefits of GLP-1 medications extend far beyond simple weight reduction. Here are some of the extended benefits that are prompting a rethinking of who can be a candidate for these therapies...

Sleep Apnea: GLP-1 therapies have been recently approved for patients with sleep apnea, offering a new therapeutic avenue for those struggling with this condition.

Fatty Liver Disease: For many patients, these medications have shown promising results in reducing, and in some cases, eliminating fatty liver disease.

Cardiovascular Health: Individuals at risk of heart-related issues can benefit from the cardiovascular advantages provided by GLP-1 treatments.

Kidney Disease: There's emerging evidence that GLP-1 drugs may also have protective effects on the kidneys, opening doors for new treatment strategies.

So, the idea that you have to be diabetic or obese to benefit from these medications is simply outdated.

Whether you're looking to improve metabolic health, manage a specific condition, or simply enjoy the benefits of a balanced lifestyle, GLP-1 therapies have a role to play — always under the careful guidance of a healthcare provider.

A Broader Perspective: Lessons from Other Medications

It might help to look at other well-known medications to appreciate how versatile treatment options can be.

Take minoxidil, for example — the star ingredient in Rogaine. Originally developed as a pill to lower high blood pressure, minoxidil found its true calling as a remedy for hair loss.

This example illustrates an important point: medications can often have more than one beneficial use, and repurposing them for different health challenges can be both ethical and effective.

Similarly, dismissing GLP-1 therapies as merely a tool for weight loss overlooks their potential to tackle a range of metabolic and cardiovascular conditions.

So next time you hear someone claim that you can't take these medications unless you fit a narrow criterion, you can confidently think, "The haters are gonna hate — but science has the last laugh! Muahaha!"

QUICK SIDE NOTE:
Another Myth/Misconception

A lot of people assume you can control the speed at which you lose weight. When I mention excess skin, or any other possible side effects that are a direct result of losing weight RAPIDLY ...
(like hair loss or muscle mass loss)

People will say, "Well, slow down! Don't be in such a rush to lose it so quickly." However, it does not work that way for those who have a large amount of weight to lose. The bigger you are, when you start your journey, the faster your body will respond.

It's like your body is eager to get the weight off, as soon as it's given the right conditions to make that possible. It's not until your body gets closer to your goal weight, that it starts to slow down & act stubborn about shedding more weight. So how fast someone loses pounds in the beginning is not really something they can help. And it has nothing to do with the GLP-1 injections. The speed is everything to do with how heavy you are when you start your journey.

Wrapping It Up

In our journey to debunk myths and address controversies, we've learned that GLP-1 medications are far more than just a shortcut to rapid weight loss.

They work by enhancing satiety, naturally curbing your appetite, and helping you make healthier food choices without the harsh effects of a starvation diet.

Moreover, their benefits extend to a range of conditions, proving that modern medicine often works in beautifully multifaceted ways.

Remember, health is not one-size-fits-all, and neither is effective treatment.

When guided by professional medical advice, GLP-1 therapies can be a powerful ally in your journey towards better health — whether you're managing diabetes, tackling sleep apnea, or simply looking to boost your overall metabolic well-being.

So, the next time you encounter naysayers, feel free to share these facts with a smile.

Embrace the science, trust the research, and let your health journey be defined by empowerment rather than misconception.

After all, innovation in healthcare is all about exploring new horizons — one well-informed step at a time!

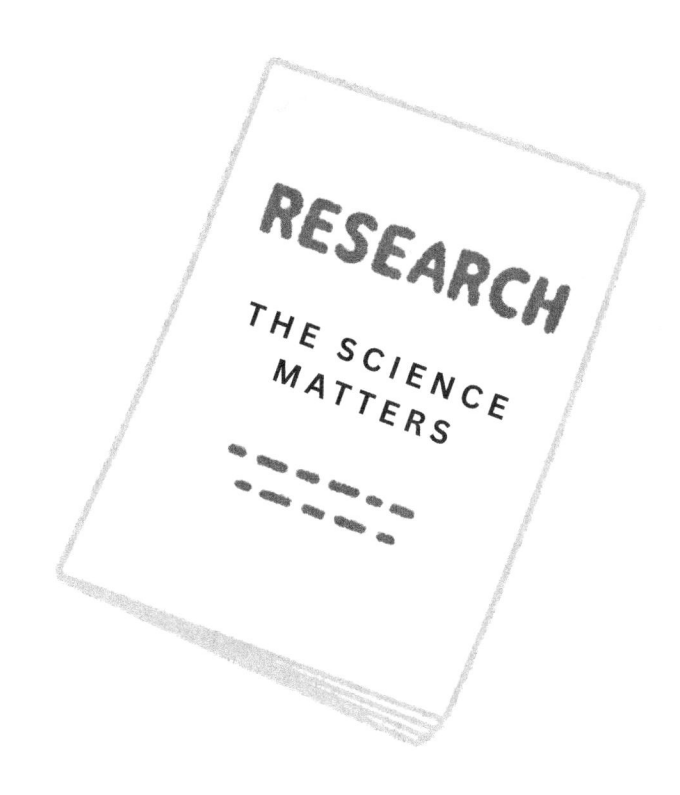

Chapter Sixteen
Side Effects & Considerations

When it comes to any medication, understanding the potential side effects is as important as knowing its benefits — and GLP-1 therapies are no exception.

We're diving deep into the world of side effects & considerations, and I'll give you practical tips for dealing with each one.

The Usual Suspects:
Common Side Effects

Starting any new medication can feel a bit like stepping into the unknown. With GLP-1 treatments, some of the more frequently encountered side effects include:

Nausea
Constipation
Fatigue
Occasional Dizziness or Light-Headedness

These symptoms tend to show up especially during the early stages of treatment.

Taming the Nausea Beast

Let's start with nausea. One of the best tricks in your arsenal? Treat it the same way a woman would handle morning sickness during pregnancy. As a mother of four, I learned a few valuable lessons on this front:

Dietary Adjustments: Small, frequent meals that are light on the stomach can do wonders. Try bland, easy-to-digest foods until you feel more settled.

Medications: If home remedies aren't cutting it, don't hesitate to talk to your doctor. They might prescribe an anti-nausea medication — the same one often recommended to pregnant women battling severe morning sickness.

Remember: a little nausea is usually a temporary side effect, and with some clever tweaks, you can keep it under control. Peppermint, Ginger, or just one or two Saltine Crackers — are effective pregnancy remedies to get rid of nausea. So sugar free mints, or peppermint tea! Eating fresh ginger as a topping on light food or in a low carb smoothie helps. Ginger ale or tea works, too!

Conquering Constipation: A Multi-Pronged Approach

Constipation is another common complaint, and trust me — it can feel like a stubborn traffic jam in your digestive system. When it hits, try tackling it from all angles...

Magnesium Supplements: Consider a daily supplement, such as magnesium glycinate or magnesium malate, both of which are gentle on your stomach.

Fiber Intake: Get plenty of fiber! Incorporate berries, Nuts & Seeds, and Green leafy vegetables into your diet to help keep things moving.

Hydration: Water is your best friend here. Keep a water bottle handy and sip throughout the day.

Physical Activity: Movement helps get things moving in more ways than one. A daily walk or a bit of light exercise can stimulate your digestive system.

Stool Softeners & Laxatives: If the above methods don't work and it's been a few days since your last bowel movement, try a gentle stool softener.

On the day it really seems necessary, a mild laxative can jump-start your system — follow it up with a stool softener for maintenance.

I speak from personal experience here — during my highest dose of semaglutide, constipation became a real nuisance. Thankfully, these steps helped me manage it effectively.

And interestingly enough, when I switched over to Tirzepatide (5mg), my constipation issues simply vanished.

It just goes to show every medication, and every person, can respond a little differently.

Full-Body Soreness & Muscle Aches:
Some of you might have experienced full-body soreness or muscle aches, particularly on the first day after an injection.

For some, this might happen every time; for others, it's just a one-off event. In my case, it was only the very first time I ever took Tirzepatide, and I've never had it happen again since.

Here's what to do if you're feeling sore...

Rest & Recovery: Take it easy. Allow your body to adjust — sometimes a day of rest is all it takes.

Gentle Movement: Light stretching, or going for an easy chill walk, can sometimes help alleviate muscle stiffness, as long as it doesn't feel like you're pushing through pain.

Remember, a bit of soreness is often your body's way of saying, "Hey, I'm working on this!" It usually fades quickly, leaving you ready to tackle your next day with renewed energy.

Dizziness & Light-Headedness: Adjusting to the New Normal

After significant weight loss, some people report feeling dizzy or light-headed — especially when they stand up too quickly. It's a common phenomenon and often related to changes in blood pressure. Here's what to do if you experience this...

Take It Slow: When rising from a seated or lying position, pause for a moment. Hold onto something if needed, and give your body time to catch up.

Monitor Your Dosage: In some cases, your doctor might suggest adjusting your dosage if your blood work indicates that your blood pressure is dipping too low.

Stay Hydrated: Hydration can help stabilize blood pressure and keep those light-headed moments at bay.

I also get a little dizzy when I stand up too fast — but usually only for a few seconds. It's a minor inconvenience, and it tends to resolve itself quickly.

Who Should Approach with Caution?

While GLP-1 medications offer a range of benefits, they aren't for everyone. For example, individuals with a history of medullary thyroid carcinoma are generally advised against using these drugs.

It's important to note, though, that this caution stems from animal studies — primarily conducted in rats — and there have been no documented cases linking these medications to thyroid issues in humans.

Additionally, discussions around risks like **gastroparesis** (delayed stomach emptying) and **pancreatitis** (inflammation of the pancreas) can sound alarming.

However, these complications are statistically rare — especially when compared to the vast number of people who safely benefit from GLP-1 therapies.

The increased media attention and widespread use of these injections can sometimes make these risks seem more common than they really are.

In reality, the more severe potential risks are actually low, and many of the reports are amplified by the sheer volume of people using these treatments worldwide. Obviously, if more & more people are taking GLP-1 injections, and it's becoming a popular medication people are eager to try... The result will be an increase in reported cases of risks coming to fruition.

Let me put it one more way. I could say I want 1/2 (half) of a pizza. Or 2/4 (two forths). Or 4/8 (four eighths)... The bigger numbers make it sound like I'm wanting more pizza than before, due to the amount of slices growing in number. But it all equaled the same amount!

The percentage didn't change, just because we increased the amount of slices the pizza got cut into. It's the same with these GLP-1 medications. It only seems like more people are suffering from the more severe risks, because the amount of people (pizza slices) taking these injections has increased.
It's still, percentage-wise, a statistically low risk.

I don't say that, to promote GLP-1s. I'm not telling you to shrug off what could be serious issues, if you were one of those unlucky few that ended up suffering from the risks. They exist! They need to be considered! You need to decide if you are willing to take that chance, for yourself. With the advice & guidance of a medical professional who can run labs on you.

However, I am also not going to fear monger you. I am not going to pretend like you should be afraid, by exaggerating the potential risks.

Everything in this book, has been about facts & personal experience. What you do with that, is completely up to you.

That's the purpose of this book. To give you insight and advice, for you to make your own educated choices. And to offer you my strategy, if you want to do what I did to lose weight!

Balancing Risks and Benefits: Trust the Science

It's all too easy to get caught up in fear-mongering narratives when it comes to new or popular medications. However, balancing these concerns with a clear understanding of scientific data is crucial.

Here are a few key takeaways:
Side effects are often temporary. Most patients find that side effects like nausea, constipation, and fatigue subside as their body adjusts.

Personal strategies can make a big difference. Simple lifestyle adjustments, dietary tweaks, and open communication with your healthcare provider can help manage most side effects.

Rare risks are just that — rare. The statistical likelihood of serious complications is low, and the benefits of GLP-1 therapies for weight management and metabolic health often far outweigh these risks.

Always consult with your healthcare provider. If you experience any side effects or have concerns about your treatment, open and honest dialogue with your doctor is key to finding the right balance for your health.

In Conclusion

Navigating the world of GLP-1 therapies doesn't have to be daunting. Yes, there are side effects to consider — from nausea and constipation to muscle aches and dizziness — but with a proactive approach and a bit of self-care, these issues can be managed effectively.

Remember, every body is unique. What works for one person may need tweaking for another, and that's why your healthcare provider is an invaluable partner on your journey.

So, whether you're a busy parent who's learned a trick or two from managing morning sickness or someone who's discovered the magic of magnesium and fiber, know that you're not alone. Embrace the process, stay informed, and keep the conversation open with your doctor. With the right strategies in place, you can navigate these temporary bumps in the road, and continue on your path to better health.

Chapter Seventeen
Hair Loss From Rapid Weightloss

The side effect I hated the most, and want you to be prepared for... The one that has me giving it, it's own chapter, instead of just listing it in the earlier side effects chapter.

I am not holding back. Im here to give it to you straight, so you can make educated choices on your own! And just like people might be worried about excess loose skin, hair loss might be something else you worry about. Or maybe you had no clue until now that THAT was a thing... Now you know!

When it comes to rapid weight loss, many individuals experience a side effect that can be as emotionally distressing as it is physically perplexing: hair loss.

It's important to understand that this **hair loss is not** a direct consequence of GLP-1 injections such as semaglutide or tirzepatide, but rather a response of the body to rapid and significant weight reduction.

Regardless of how the weight is lost — whether through dietary changes, exercise, surgery, or pharmacotherapy — the body can perceive this rapid change as a form of trauma, triggering a phenomenon known as telogen effluvium.

Telogen effluvium is a well-documented condition in which a large number of hair follicles prematurely enter the resting phase, eventually leading to noticeable shedding.

Typically, the hair loss does not occur immediately; it generally begins around three months after the body experiences what it recognizes as a traumatic event. In the context of rapid weight loss, the stress imposed on the body disrupts the natural hair growth cycle.

The follicles that would normally continue to grow are signaled to stop, and after a delay of about three months, those hairs begin to shed. This delay is a hallmark of the condition: the hair that falls out corresponds to the period of rapid weight loss that occurred three months prior.

The phenomenon is a classic example of how the body prioritizes survival over aesthetic concerns when it is under stress.

When significant weight is lost quickly, the body is suddenly faced with a drastic change in energy reserves, and it responds by reallocating resources away from non-essential functions — such as hair growth — to more critical systems.

While this is an adaptive mechanism designed to protect vital organs and maintain overall metabolic stability, it comes at the cost of temporary hair loss.

Fortunately, this type of hair loss is temporary. As the rate of weight loss slows and the body begins to settle into its new metabolic state, the hair follicles eventually exit the resting phase and re-enter the active growth cycle.

New hair will start to emerge, and over time, most individuals will see their hair return to its former density and vitality. The duration of the shedding period can vary; it will continue for as long as the body experiences rapid weight loss, but once that phase stabilizes, the process of regrowth usually begins and continues progressively.

There are several strategies that can help mitigate the severity of hair loss during this period. Although it is a natural response to rapid weight loss, adopting certain practices can support the health of your hair and scalp during this challenging time.

For instance, natural remedies such as rosemary oil have been traditionally used to stimulate blood flow to the scalp, potentially supporting hair growth.

Additionally, the use of DHT shampoo and conditioner can be beneficial for those who are concerned about hormone-related hair thinning, while minoxidil — a topical treatment well-known for its hair regrowth properties — may be recommended by healthcare providers to encourage regrowth in susceptible areas.

It should be noted, however, that if you start using minoxidil, you will be stuck having to use it daily, for life! Because whatever hair you gained from using minoxidil, will fall out with a vengeance if you ever stop using it daily. So just remember that choosing minoxidil is choosing a life-long daily commitment.

Also, the physical treatment of your hair matters too. Opting for gentle brushes that reduce friction, and sleeping with a satin bonnet, can help prevent additional breakage and mechanical damage to fragile hair strands.

Beyond these external measures, ensuring that your body receives the proper nutrients is critical.

Maintaining an adequate intake of essential vitamins and minerals, particularly iron, is paramount because deficiencies can exacerbate hair loss.

It is important, however, to adhere to the recommended daily value of iron, to avoid any potential side effects from over-supplementation. It is possible to overdose iron. So be careful about taking the correct daily amount.

Regular scalp massages and emerging treatments like red light therapy may also promote a healthier scalp environment and encourage hair follicle activity.

While these methods can help slow down and lessen the amount of hair lost, it is essential to approach the situation with a sense of perspective.

The hair loss experienced as a result of rapid weight loss is generally reversible. As your body acclimates to its new state, and the rapid weight reduction phase comes to a close, the stress signals that once disrupted the hair growth cycle diminish, and the hair begins to grow back.

This regrowth process, while it may take several months, ultimately restores your hair to its natural state.

Understanding that hair loss in the context of rapid weight loss is a physiological response, rather than a permanent change can provide comfort.

It's a reminder that our bodies have intricate systems designed to protect us in times of stress — even if those protective mechanisms sometimes lead to undesirable temporary outcomes.

It's also a call to be patient and gentle with yourself during the transition. Because hair loss can feel rough.

Monitoring your overall health, consulting with healthcare providers, and employing supportive hair care practices can all contribute to a smoother recovery.

In conclusion, while the rapid weight loss achieved through GLP-1 injections or other methods can trigger temporary hair shedding, this response is not a direct consequence of the medications themselves, but rather a natural, albeit distressing, reaction of the body to significant change.

With time, appropriate care, and a balanced approach to both your overall health and hair care regimen, your hair will eventually regain its strength and fullness.

This process, though challenging in the short term, underscores the resilience of the human body and its remarkable ability to adapt and heal over time.

Chapter Eighteen
Emotional Challenges in Weight Loss

Facing emotional challenges during weight loss can feel like an uphill battle, with emotions running high and often getting the best of us.

The journey isn't just about swapping donuts for salads or hitting the gym more often; it's a complex path that involves understanding our relationship with food and emotions.

Emotional hurdles can sneak in and sabotage even the best-laid plans, leaving us feeling defeated before we've truly begun. It's important to recognize these emotional undercurrents as they play a crucial role in shaping our habits and decision-making processes.

Our minds can be our biggest allies or fiercest foes, influencing us to seek comfort in food when times get tough. But just as a tailor mends a torn seam with precision and care, so too can we adjust our mindsets, addressing these emotional barriers with empathy and strategies that nurture long-lasting change.

This chapter delves into the intricate dance between emotions and eating, dissecting how stress, boredom, and sadness trigger emotional eating.

It guides you in differentiating between emotional hunger and physical hunger, helping you recognize the subtle signals your body sends. You'll explore the underlying triggers of emotional eating and learn practical ways to develop healthier coping mechanisms.

Whether it's through mindfulness, exercise, or simply talking things out, the chapter provides actionable insights to foster a more balanced emotional state. With the right tools and perspective shifts, breaking free from the cycle of emotional eating becomes not only possible but empowering.

By the end, you'll understand how to build a supportive environment and approach each meal with mindfulness, creating a harmonious relationship with food that transcends momentary cravings and fosters a healthier, more fulfilling lifestyle.

Understanding Emotional Eating

Emotional eating is a common behavior where individuals turn to food for comfort, especially during times of stress or emotional turmoil, rather than because they are physically hungry. It's like seeking solace in a bowl of ice cream after a bad day at work, turning to snacks when feeling bored, or indulging in a heavy meal when overwhelmed by sadness.

This habit diverges from physical hunger, which is our body's natural signal that it needs nourishment for energy and sustenance.

Recognizing the triggers that lead to emotional eating is crucial because awareness is the first step towards change. Stress is a major factor; many people find themselves reaching for comforting foods when they feel anxious or pressured.

Similarly, boredom can lead to unnecessary snacking just to fill the time.

Sadness or loneliness can also drive people to seek warmth in their favorite meals. Identifying these emotions as they arise helps to break the cycle of emotional eating. By pinpointing specific triggers, you can start to address them with strategies that don't involve food.

Differentiating between emotional hunger and physical hunger is another important aspect of combating emotional eating. Physical hunger develops gradually and can be satisfied with any type of food; it's accompanied by physiological signals like stomach growling.

Emotional hunger, on the other hand, comes on suddenly. It often craves specific comfort foods — typically those high in sugar, fat, or salt — and isn't easily satisfied.

Emotional hunger persists even after you're full, whereas physical hunger dissipates once you've eaten enough. Understanding these distinctions can guide healthier food choices and help reduce reliance on food as an emotional crutch.

Developing alternative coping mechanisms is essential for emotional regulation. Exercise is a powerful tool in this regard.

Physical activity releases endorphins, the brain's feel-good chemicals, which naturally elevate your mood and reduce stress.

Even a short walk, yoga session, or dance break can help clear your mind and alleviate negative emotions without turning to food for relief.

Other strategies might include engaging in hobbies you enjoy, practicing mindfulness or meditation, or talking through your feelings with a friend or therapist.

These activities provide healthier outlets for managing emotions, reducing the dependence on food for emotional support.

Guidelines for overcoming emotional eating involve practical steps to establish a healthier relationship with food and emotions. For instance, keeping a food journal can help you track what's driving your eating patterns.

When you notice a craving, pause and ask yourself if it's physical or emotional hunger — this simple act of reflection can prevent impulsive eating.

Setting up regular meal times and planning meals in advance can also contribute to better eating habits, reducing the likelihood of using food as an emotional response.

Another key guideline involves creating an environment that supports positive choices. Stock your kitchen with healthy snack options and keep tempting indulgences out of sight.

When emotional urges strike, try drinking a glass of water or distracting yourself with a non-food-related activity before deciding whether to eat.

Additionally, cultivating self-compassion plays a critical role in addressing emotional eating. Be kind to yourself and recognize that setbacks happen. Viewing them as opportunities for learning and growth, can help build resilience and foster long-term change.

Building healthy relationships with food involves changing how we perceive and interact with what we eat. It's about listening to our bodies and enjoying food mindfully, taking pleasure in flavors and textures without guilt.

Practicing mindful eating means being present during meals, savoring each bite, and paying attention to how different foods make you feel.

This practice encourages more conscious choices and diminishes the automatic nature of emotional eating.

Furthermore, building a supportive network can reinforce healthier habits. Sharing experiences with friends or joining a support group provides accountability and encouragement, reminding you that you're not alone on this journey.

Discussing challenges and successes with others can offer new perspectives and strategies for transforming your relationship with food.

Dealing with Body Image Perceptions

Body image is an individual's perception and feeling about their own body, which can greatly affect mental health and weight loss efforts.

At its core, body image is deeply tied to cultural standards and media portrayals. Society's depiction of the "ideal" body, often through advertisements, films, and social media, sets a standard that many individuals feel pressured to meet.

This pressure can distort one's self-perception, leading them to judge themselves harshly if they don't align with these external ideals.

The repercussions of a negative body image are significant. When individuals frequently perceive their bodies negatively, it often results in low self-esteem, impacting various aspects of life, including relationships and professional endeavors.

In the context of a weight loss journey, poor self-esteem can be particularly detrimental.

Those struggling with weight may already face challenges with motivation and resilience, and adding a layer of negative body perception can intensify feelings of inadequacy, making it harder to maintain positive momentum toward weight goals.

However, addressing this issue isn't just about identifying the problem — it's about cultivating solutions, such as practicing self-compassion and engaging in positive self-talk.

Self-compassion involves treating oneself with kindness and understanding, especially when encountering personal failures or setbacks.

By acknowledging that everyone has imperfections and that it's okay to have shortcomings, individuals can start to foster a healthier relationship with their bodies. Positive self-talk complements this by encouraging affirmations and supportive dialogue within oneself.

Rather than focusing on perceived flaws, emphasizing strengths and expressing gratitude for what our bodies can do is crucial.

For example, instead of fixating on weight gain, one might appreciate their body's strength and endurance or celebrate small victories in fitness or healthy eating.

Questioning societal norms surrounding body image plays an essential role in reshaping self-perceptions.

Many societal standards are unrealistic or based on outdated stereotypes that don't reflect diverse and natural body types.

Challenging these norms involves critically assessing the images we consume and recognizing that these portrayals aren't definitive paths to beauty or success.

This critical approach provides liberation from unhealthy stereotypes, allowing individuals to embrace their unique attributes without comparing themselves to unrealistic benchmarks.

By shifting focus away from fitting societal molds to appreciating individuality, people find greater acceptance and contentment with their bodies.

A guideline worth mentioning for cultivating a positive body image involves integrating self-compassion practices into daily routines.

An individual might set aside a few moments each day to reflect on positive affirmations, celebrate achievements, and practice gratitude towards their body. This intentional practice can gradually shift perceptions and reinforce a supportive internal narrative that outshines damaging external influences.

Coping with Self-Doubt and Anxiety

Overcoming self-doubt and anxiety during a weight loss journey can be a challenging task. It's like standing at the base of a mountain you're about to climb, feeling both excitement and trepidation.

One way to start addressing these emotional hurdles is by identifying the sources of your self-doubt. Often, fear of failure looms large in our minds, whispering doubts about our ability to succeed.

Recognizing that this fear exists is the first step towards addressing it. Consider keeping a journal where you note down triggers or moments when self-doubt hits hardest.

This awareness doesn't just help map out your emotional landscape but also paves the way for strategies designed to counteract these feelings.

Once you have a handle on what might be fueling your self-doubt, turning to mindfulness techniques can be incredibly beneficial.

Mindfulness is about being present in the moment, acknowledging your thoughts without judgment, and letting them pass.

Techniques such as deep breathing, meditation, or even yoga can help reduce anxiety significantly.
Imagine starting your day with a few minutes of focused breathing — this small act can foster a sense of calm and control that sets a positive tone for the rest of the day.

Regular practice can result in long-term benefits, such as reduced stress levels and improved emotional resilience, which are crucial during the ups and downs of a weight loss journey.

The prospect of failure can be daunting and may lead many to shy away from their goals entirely. However, embracing failure as a learning opportunity rather than a setback can transform your outlook.

Each stumble is not the end but a chance to gather insights and strengthen resolve. For instance, if you have an off-day with your diet or exercise routine, instead of berating yourself, analyze what happened and how different choices might lead to better outcomes.

This shift in perspective helps build resilience and fosters a stronger commitment to your goals. Remember, every successful person has faced failures along the way; it's how they learned and grew that made the difference.

Practicing self-compassion is another essential guideline. Treating yourself with kindness during tough times is crucial. When negative thoughts creep in, counter them with positive affirmations. Remind yourself that progress, not perfection, is the real goal.

Self-compassion provides an emotional buffer against the sting of self-doubt and reinforces the belief that you are worthy of achieving your aspirations, regardless of hiccups along the way.

On top of personal strategies, seeking support from others can offer immense relief. Isolation can exacerbate feelings of self-doubt and anxiety, but connecting with supportive friends, family, or weight loss communities can make the journey a little less lonely.

Sharing experiences with others who understand your struggles can provide encouragement and motivation. Imagine having a friend who cheers you on after each little victory or offers words of wisdom when you're feeling low — that kind of support is invaluable.

participating in group activities or engaging in online forums dedicated to weight loss can provide additional layers of support.

Many find comfort in knowing they aren't alone in their experiences, and hearing others' stories of triumph over similar challenges can reignite one's own determination.

These social connections can also introduce you to new coping mechanisms and insights that you might not have considered on your own.

Incorporating these strategies into your daily routine might seem overwhelming at first, but remember, change takes time.

Start small, perhaps integrating one technique at a time until it becomes a natural part of your life.

Overcoming self-doubt and anxiety is not about eradicating these feelings entirely but managing and reducing their impact on your weight loss journey.

As you implement these strategies, you'll likely notice a shift in how you approach obstacles — not just in terms of weight loss but in various aspects of life. Your confidence will grow, along with a renewed belief in your capabilities.

Navigating the emotional hurdles in a weight loss journey is no small feat, but recognizing these challenges is the first stride towards overcoming them.

We've explored how emotions like stress, boredom, and sadness often lead to emotional eating, which can derail our efforts even before we realize it.

By identifying triggers and differentiating between emotional hunger and physical hunger, you can start breaking the cycle.

This chapter shed light on developing alternative coping mechanisms, such as exercise, mindfulness, and engaging in hobbies to manage emotions healthily. These strategies help foster a better relationship with food and build resilience along the journey.

As we wrap up this discussion, it's important to remember that setbacks are not failures; they're part of the process. Embracing self-compassion and building supportive networks can keep you grounded and motivated.

Whether it's journaling to track progress or leaning on friends and family for encouragement, every step you take signifies growth.

Remember, change doesn't happen overnight — it's about gradual shifts towards healthier habits and mindsets.

With patience and persistence, you're creating a foundation for lasting change and a more positive approach to your unique weight loss path.

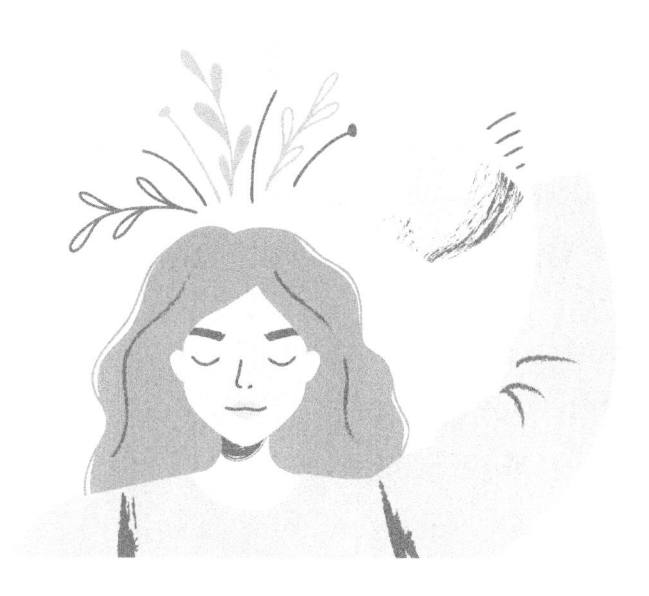

Chapter Nineteen
Societal Stigma and Obesity

Societal stigma and obesity are deeply intertwined, affecting many aspects of life for those living with weight challenges.

Society's perception of body size has fluctuated throughout history, swinging from admiration in ancient times to criticism in more modern eras. Understanding how these perceptions have evolved helps us unravel the complex web of stigma that exists today.

This chapter takes a journey through time, examining how cultural narratives about obesity have been shaped by economic, social, and medical developments.

By exploring these shifts, we can start to see how past beliefs influence current attitudes and contribute to the pervasive stigma faced by individuals with obesity.

As we delve deeper, this chapter will guide readers through various societal impacts of obesity stigma, including its effects on mental health and healthcare access.

You'll learn about how weight-related discrimination negatively impacts individuals' self-esteem, mental well-being, and their interactions within healthcare environments.

The historical context sets the stage for understanding today's biases, while stories from personal experiences connect these themes to real-world consequences.

Additionally, the chapter will explore media representations and public policies that either challenge or perpetuate stereotypes about obesity.
With an emphasis on inclusive practices and shifting narratives, this exploration seeks to promote empathy and highlight the importance of supportive communities in dismantling harmful stigmas

Historical Context of Obesity Stigma

Throughout history, the way societies perceive obesity has shaped today's attitudes and societal norms. It's fascinating to look back at ancient times when being plump was often seen as a sign of wealth and prosperity. In some cultures, it symbolized abundance and health, as only the affluent could afford excess food.

For instance, in ancient Greece, full-bodied figures were depicted in art, suggesting that they enjoyed a positive status.

Similarly, during the Renaissance in Europe, voluptuousness was celebrated in artwork, reflecting an appreciation for fuller forms.

However, not every society viewed obesity positively. In some periods, such as during the rise of industrialization, leaner bodies came to represent efficiency and hard work.

This shift mirrored changing economic realities, where physical labor and productivity became highly valued. As the world evolved, these varying cultural perceptions contributed to a patchwork of beliefs about body size, influencing how we understand obesity today.

Misconceptions about obesity have long fueled stigma, often perceiving it as a personal failure or lack of willpower. This view overlooks the complex interplay of genetics, environment, and psychological factors that contribute to weight.

The notion that sheer determination alone can manage obesity is not only incorrect but also harmful. Such misconceptions are rooted in outdated ideas that ignore scientific advancements in understanding metabolism and body composition.

The advent of medical definitions and categories has played a significant role in shaping perceptions over the years. In the past, medical practitioners focused primarily on visible signs rather than underlying causes.

Over time, however, the medical field has shifted towards more nuanced understandings, recognizing obesity as a multifaceted health issue.

Modern medical definitions emphasize body mass index (BMI) and other health indicators, factoring in individual differences rather than relying solely on appearance.

This evolution highlights the growing awareness of obesity as more than just excess weight, paving the path for better healthcare approaches.

Legislation and public policies offer another lens through which to view societal attitudes toward obesity.

Laws and regulations often mirror the prevailing values and biases of their time. Historically, legislation has sometimes reinforced negative stereotypes by focusing solely on weight loss initiatives without addressing broader systemic issues.

However, there have been efforts to promote inclusivity and understanding. Some countries have introduced policies that recognize obesity as a chronic condition, aiming to reduce discrimination and encourage supportive health services.

These legal frameworks reflect a gradual shift towards recognizing obesity's complexity, though challenges remain.

Effects of Stigma on Mental Health

Weight-related stigma is not just a matter of hurt feelings — it has profound consequences for mental health and overall well-being.

One of the most immediate impacts of societal stigma is a heightened sense of anxiety. Individuals suffering from obesity often feel under constant scrutiny, fearing judgment at every turn.

This relentless worry can escalate into chronic anxiety, where every social interaction feels like a potential confrontation or an occasion for ridicule.

Depression is another common mental health issue linked to weight stigma. The feeling of being devalued or dismissed by society can create a pervasive sense of hopelessness.

Depression creeps in when individuals internalize the negative messages they receive about their body, leading them to believe that they are somehow less worthy.

Their self-worth becomes entangled with societal perceptions, making happiness seem elusive.

Low self-esteem goes hand in hand with these mental health challenges. Constant exposure to derogatory remarks and stigmatizing attitudes can shatter confidence, making individuals feel inferior.

The reflection in the mirror becomes distorted by societal negativity, turning self-image into an enemy rather than a source of empowerment.

Delving deeper, internalized stigma adds another layer of complexity. Many people begin to accept harsh societal judgments as truths. Struggling with weight becomes not just a physical battle, but a psychological one.

They may believe they deserve the stigma because they haven't met society's narrow standards of beauty or health. This internalization manifests in unhealthy coping mechanisms.

Emotional eating might become a go-to solution for battling stress or sadness, creating a vicious cycle of weight gain and further stigma.

To combat these harmful beliefs, it's crucial to break this cycle. Seeking support from therapists or support groups who specialize in body positivity can be transformative. These resources provide safe spaces where individuals can rebuild their self-esteem and challenge ingrained beliefs.

It's also beneficial to practice self-compassion. Reminding oneself that everyone deserves kindness, regardless of size, can gradually shift ingrained perspectives.

The stigma surrounding obesity also creates substantial barriers to seeking necessary healthcare. Many avoid doctor visits out of fear of being judged, criticized, or receiving unsolicited advice about their weight.

The idea of stepping into a medical office can evoke dread, knowing the focus often skews towards weight rather than the actual health issue at hand. This avoidance can lead to untreated conditions and worsening health outcomes.

Healthcare professionals have a responsibility to cultivate an environment free from bias. It's essential for them to communicate openly, focusing on the individual's holistic health rather than just numbers on a scale.

Educating themselves about the impact of stigma can change interactions dramatically, ensuring that patients feel respected and heard.

On a broader scale, obese individuals face social ramifications that extend beyond personal relationships. Bullying is a troubling reality for many, starting from childhood and sometimes persisting into adulthood.

The emotional scars left by bullying can linger long after the taunts cease, affecting interpersonal relationships and trust.

Isolation is a related consequence. Feeling unloved or unwanted can drive people away from social gatherings, limiting opportunities for forming meaningful connections.

The assumption that they won't fit in or will be targeted can keep individuals socially confined, amplifying feelings of loneliness.

It takes a community effort to dismantle these barriers. We can normalize diverse body types and challenge outdated stereotypes through active participation in advocacy efforts or simply by having open conversations.

By collectively condemning acts of bullying and ostracism, we help create inclusive environments where all individuals are valued.

Education plays a critical role in this process. Teaching empathy and understanding from a young age can fundamentally alter perceptions.

Schools and communities can promote programs that highlight the importance of diversity and acceptance, instilling values that counteract stigma before it takes root.

Media Representations of Body Image

The way media portrays obesity has a significant impact on societal attitudes and the stigma surrounding the condition. Films and television often perpetuate stereotypes of obese individuals, usually characterizing them in negative or comedic roles that reinforce harmful perceptions.

These portrayals can influence viewers' understanding of obesity, leading to oversimplified and judgmental views about people who are overweight.

For example, in many movies and shows, characters with larger body sizes are frequently depicted as lazy, undisciplined, or lacking self-control.

This messaging is not just damaging but misleading, as it fails to consider the complex factors contributing to obesity, such as genetics and socioeconomic status.

Such representations make it challenging for society to view obesity from a compassionate perspective, supporting individuals rather than blaming them.

In the realm of advertising, the glorification of thinness is prevalent. Primarily, unrealistic body proportions that are not usually natural, and would require cosmetic surgery to even achieve. The media consistently pushes an idealized images of what one should look like, that are often unattainable for most.

Advertisements tend to valorize products promising weight loss success or miraculous transformations, that are also usually full of crap & fake! Even with GLP-1 medications, you have companies & weight loss "clinics" out there selling fake compound versions of the shots, to scam people out of money!
(Always be careful of that! Always make sure the GLP-1 medicine you get is real, before taking it, if you go the compound route)

Some (not all) fitness and diet industries capitalize on this, by promoting "quick-fix solutions" instead of healthy long-term lifestyle changes, and contribute to a culture that shames those living with obesity, as if it should of been easy to lose weight.

However, there is growing recognition and effort to shift these narratives through various initiatives. Increasingly, campaigns and programs are aiming to promote body diversity and challenge traditional beauty standards.

Brands and media outlets are beginning to feature a broader range of body types, emphasizing that beauty comes in all shapes and sizes.

This positive representation is essential in reducing stigma associated with obesity.

Guidelines for advertisers to follow can help foster this movement. A commitment to featuring diverse body types in campaigns is awesome, but using language that promotes health (not just appearance) are some steps that can transform the media landscape.

These efforts can ultimately encourage inclusivity and respect for all individuals, while still promoting health.

Social media is another arena where societal stigma around obesity plays out. It serves a dual role — while it can perpetuate unhealthy ideals, it also provides a platform for advocacy and support for body positivity.

On the negative side, social media is rife with influencers promoting unrealistic standards of beauty that many try to emulate. Or TOXIC pretend Body Positivity.

Whether it's through heavily edited photos perpetuating harmful ideas of how everyone should look. Or through "Fat-Fluencers" (their choice of name) who shame the other end of the scale, trying to promote being obese -- under the fake pretense of "Body Positivity"

You aren't body possitive when you shame people for being normal weight, or shame someone for wanting to lose weight for their health. "Health at Every Size" is total bullcrap! Sorry, but being mobidly obese is bad for your health. You deserve to be loved & respected, but should be encouraged to get healthy.

Social media also offers communities where people can connect, share their stories, and find solace in shared experiences. So there's good to social media, as well.

Platforms are being used increasingly for non-toxic body positivity movements, that genuinely celebrate **all body types** and challenge the stigmas associated with being overweight. Shedding light on how complex obesity is.

By showcasing real people and their journeys toward self-acceptance, these spaces provide much-needed support and inspiration for those affected by societal pressures.

Guiding users on how to engage responsibly with social media content related to body image is crucial. Encouraging critical thinking about what is consumed online, following diverse accounts, and engaging in conversations about health and wellness, rather than just appearance, can cultivate a more balanced online experience.

As we've seen, societal attitudes towards obesity have deep roots in history and culture.

From ancient times when a fuller figure was often admired to periods where thinness became the norm, cultural shifts have shaped the way we view body size today.

Unfortunately, this has led to significant stigma around obesity, with harmful misconceptions painting it as a personal failure rather than recognizing the complex factors involved.

This chapter highlighted how legislation, media, and society at large contribute to these perceptions, often ignoring scientific advancements that offer a more compassionate understanding of obesity.

But it's not all grim news! There are efforts underway to challenge and change these outdated views.

Healthcare professionals are increasingly adopting approaches that consider the individual beyond just numbers on a scale, and media outlets are beginning to celebrate body diversity.

For those affected by stigma, finding supportive communities and resources can be empowering.

By promoting **REAL** body positivity, we can work towards a future where everyone, regardless of size, feels valued and respected. While still encouraging getting healthy!

Let's continue to shift the narrative and break the cycle of stigma for a healthier, kinder world.

Chapter Twenty
Lessons Learned From Challenges

Beginning a journey with GLP-1 medications often presents several hurdles that require resilience and problem-solving strategies to overcome.

At the outset, individuals may face challenges such as adjusting to new routines or managing side effects. These initial setbacks can feel overwhelming, but they serve as critical learning opportunities.

For instance, some people experience nausea or diminished appetite when they first start their treatment. Understanding that these symptoms are common and typically decrease over time can help reduce anxiety.

Consulting with healthcare providers for personalized advice can smooth this transition, providing reassurance and helping to adjust dosage if necessary.
Resilience becomes an invaluable trait during these early phases. Drawing from support networks — be it family, friends, or online communities — can foster a sense of belonging and understanding.

Sharing experiences allows individuals to learn from others who have successfully navigated similar issues.

The key is not to view these initial problems as failures but as part of the learning curve in adapting to a new lifestyle aided by medication.

Creating an open dialogue with health professionals also plays a crucial role, enabling adjustments and offering tailored strategies that align more closely with individual needs.

As weight loss progresses, many encounter plateaus, which can dampen motivation. It's important to recognize that these pauses in weight loss are normal and temporary.

Here, flexibility in approach is essential. Sometimes altering exercise routines or tweaking dietary habits can reignite progress. Incorporating varied physical activities can both break monotony and challenge the body in new ways, helping to overcome stagnation.

Setting incremental goals rather than focusing solely on long-term objectives helps maintain motivation.

Celebrating small victories along the way reinforces positive behaviors and provides a consistent morale boost.

Motivational techniques are equally valuable during these plateau periods.

Visualizing end goals, practicing mindfulness, or even keeping a journal of daily achievements can reinforce one's commitment.

Engaging in group activities or finding a workout buddy can inject social elements into the routine, making it more enjoyable and less isolating.

These techniques not only help traverse the plateau phase but also encourage a shift in mindset — from viewing weight loss as a linear journey to embracing its complexities as natural parts of the process.

Mental health struggles often accompany the weight-loss journey, underscoring the importance of addressing psychological challenges head-on.

Emotional well-being is closely tied to physical health;

therefore, opening a dialogue about common mental health issues encountered during weight loss is crucial. Stress, depression, or anxiety can arise from changes in body image, societal pressures, or personal expectations. Recognizing these feelings as valid and seeking professional mental health support can aid in managing them effectively.

Coping mechanisms such as therapy, meditation, and stress management techniques can provide relief and promote mental resilience.

Cognitive-behavioral therapy (CBT) offers tools for restructuring negative thought patterns, fostering a more balanced perspective on personal progress.

Additionally, participating in support groups can offer emotional validation and shared experiences, reminding individuals they are not alone in their struggles.

Acknowledging and attending to mental health is not just supportive — it's a vital component of a holistic approach to weight management.

Understanding relapse as a natural part of the journey is another significant aspect. Many experience moments of setback, whether through regained weight or lapses in medication adherence.

Importantly, these should be seen not as failures but as opportunities for growth and learning. Normalizing relapse helps remove stigma and fosters a kinder self-perspective.

It's crucial to analyze any factors contributing to the setback: Was there a particular trigger? Did certain stressors lead to old habits resurfacing?

Regaining momentum involves setting realistic short-term goals and leaning into the supportive structures previously established. Small, achievable steps can rebuild confidence incrementally.

Sharing these experiences candidly with healthcare providers can result in actionable insights tailored to prevent future relapse. Emphasizing the cyclical nature of success and failure allows individuals to approach their journey with greater empathy towards themselves.

Overcoming Personal Obstacles

Overcoming the societal stigma surrounding weight is a journey fraught with internal and external challenges.

Many individuals who embark on weight loss journeys using GLP-1 medications often face prejudices that can undermine their self-worth.

In our society, there's a pervasive tendency to judge others based solely on appearance, leading to unwarranted assumptions about personal habits and character.

One of the most effective ways to navigate these stigmas is by cultivating strong self-confidence — a process rooted in understanding one's worth beyond physical attributes.

By prioritizing personal goals over societal judgments, individuals can shift their focus from external expectations to self-defined success. This mindset fosters resilience and empowers individuals to pursue their health objectives without being derailed by negativity.

Addressing self-doubt and maintaining motivation can be daunting, but it's crucial for those navigating weight loss journeys.

Self-doubt often creeps in subtly, fueled by past failures or perceived inadequacies. To combat this, individuals should establish a positive inner dialogue, treating themselves with kindness and patience as they would a cherished friend.

Utilizing motivational strategies like setting short-term goals and celebrating small victories can create a sense of momentum.

It's also beneficial to visualize long-term achievements, reinforcing the belief that change is not only possible but attainable. A practical guideline here involves developing a daily affirmation practice or journaling about positive experiences to build a foundation of self-belief.

Lifestyle changes play a pivotal role in achieving sustained weight loss beyond merely relying on medication. Incorporating healthier habits — such as balanced nutrition, regular physical activity, and adequate sleep — can enhance the effectiveness of treatments like GLP-1.

Chapter Twenty-One
Economic and Healthcare Implications

As GLP-1 therapies become increasingly mainstream, their economic and healthcare implications are gaining prominence. The widespread adoption of these medications is affecting healthcare systems, insurance models, and patient access worldwide. We should also consider the potential cost-effectiveness and long-term savings associated with reduced comorbidities, alongside the challenges posed by high medication costs, and varying access across regions within the United States.

Impact on Healthcare Systems Shift in Treatment

Paradigms: The success of GLP-1 therapies is prompting a reevaluation of traditional treatment approaches for obesity and type 2 diabetes. With proven efficacy in weight loss and metabolic control, these medications are being integrated into standard care protocols.

Reduction in Comorbidities: By effectively reducing weight and improving metabolic parameters, GLP-1 medications have the potential to lower the incidence of associated comorbidities such as cardiovascular disease, type 2 diabetes complications, and certain cancers. This can translate into fewer hospitalizations and a reduced burden on healthcare resources.

Long-Term Savings: Economic models suggest that, despite the upfront costs of these medications, the long-term savings from reduced comorbidity management and fewer invasive procedures (such as bariatric surgery) could be substantial. Studies have projected significant cost offsets due to the prevention of costly chronic conditions.

Insurance Models and Cost-Effectiveness

Reimbursement Challenges: Initially, many insurance providers were hesitant to cover these medications due to their high cost. However, as clinical evidence accumulates, there is a growing recognition of their cost-effectiveness.

Value-Based Pricing: Payers are increasingly considering value- based pricing models where reimbursement is tied to the achievement of clinical outcomes such as weight loss and improved glycemic control. This aligns the interests of manufacturers, providers, and patients.

Economic Evaluations: Health economics studies have reported favorable cost-effectiveness ratios for GLP-1 therapies, especially when considering the downstream savings from reduced healthcare utilization. For example, a reduction in the need for diabetes medications or cardiovascular interventions can help justify the investment in these therapies.

This is a hard topic to discuss, because my view on insurance is a political one that not many folks around me (living in a red state) agree with.
But all our government has to do, if they were not so damn corrupt, is put a price cap on these GLP-1 medications. We don't even have to discuss universal healthcare. All we need is legistlation passed into law, where the government says pharmaceutical companies are no longer allowed to mark up drug prices past a certain percentage worth of profits. They can make their profits and still be rich, without price-gouging and robbing us blind, for all they can get.

Other governments outside the US have price capped what GLP-1s can cost in their countries. And the difference is huge.

Instead of the $1,200 to $1,300 that **ONE MONTH** of injections can cost in the United States...
It's closer to $300 or $500 on average in other countries, per month. Depending on which country, of course, but still...
That is a lot less, because their governments refuse to pay more than they have to.

I understand insurance is a hot topic, but even without the discussion of insurance, we could at the very least - get a price cap, to help make it more affordable.

And for the record, if it was more affordable, insurance companies would not be so "iffy" about whether or not they are willing to cover it for patients in need. Lowering the costs helps increase the likelihood of getting coverage.

To briefly summarize, the economic and healthcare implications of GLP-1 medications are multifaceted and far-reaching.

While their high upfront cost poses challenges, the long-term benefits — both clinical and economic — suggest that these therapies may ultimately reduce the overall burden of obesity-related diseases. By fostering a shift toward value-based care and implementing policies that enhance access, healthcare systems can harness the full potential of GLP-1 therapies to improve public health outcomes on a global scale.

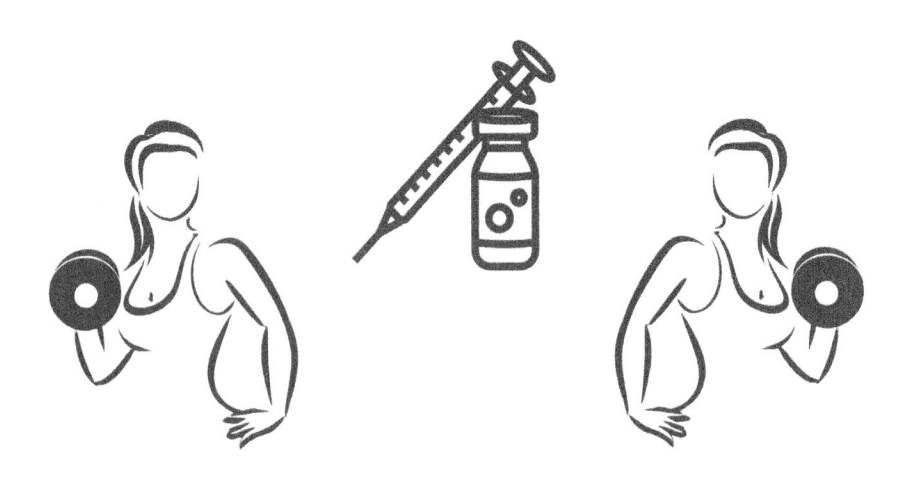

Chapter Twenty-Two
Clinical Trials & Evidence-Based Outcomes

This chapter examines the clinical research that has shaped the current understanding and usage of GLP-1 therapies in weight management and metabolic health. By reviewing major clinical studies, we will explore the data on weight loss, metabolic improvements, long-term safety, and quality of life. In addition, we discuss ongoing research efforts that continue to refine our approach to these treatments.

Major Clinical Trials Shaping GLP-1 Therapy
Semaglutide Trials – The STEP Program

STEP 1 Trial
- **Design:** A randomized, double-blind, placebo-controlled trial involving adults with overweight or obesity.
- **Intervention:** Participants received once-weekly semaglutide 2.4 mg.

Key Outcomes:
- **Weight Loss:** Participants experienced an average weight loss of approximately 15% of their initial body weight.

- **Metabolic Improvements:** Significant reductions in waist circumference and improvements in glycemic control were observed.
- **Quality of Life:** Enhanced physical functioning and self-perception were reported through validated quality-of-life questionnaires.
- **Significance:** This study provided robust evidence for the efficacy of semaglutide as a weight-loss agent, influencing regulatory approvals and clinical guidelines.

STEP 2 and STEP 3 Trials

- **Focus:** These studies further examined semaglutide's benefits in populations with type 2 diabetes and evaluated additional lifestyle intervention components.
- **Results:** Confirmed the dual benefits of improved glycemic control alongside weight reduction, reinforcing the role of semaglutide in managing metabolic syndrome components.

Tirzepatide Trials – The SURPASS Program
SURPASS-2 Trial

- **Design:** A randomized, controlled trial comparing tirzepatide with standard diabetes care.
- **Intervention:** Tirzepatide, a dual GIP and GLP-1 receptor agonist, was administered once weekly.

Key Outcomes:

- **Weight Loss:** Patients achieved up to 20% weight loss in some arms of the study, surpassing traditional GLP-1 receptor agonist outcomes.
- **Glycemic Control:** Marked reductions in HbA1c levels were observed, often leading to near-normal glycemic ranges.
- **Safety Profile:** Adverse events were predominantly gastrointestinal and transient, consistent with expectations.
- **Significance:** SURPASS-2 highlights the potential for enhanced weight loss and metabolic benefits with dual agonism, positioning tirzepatide as a promising next-generation therapy.

Long-Term Safety and Quality of Life Studies
Extended Follow-Up Studies

- **Duration:** Many studies have followed patients for 68 weeks or more.
- **Findings:**
    - Safety: The incidence of severe adverse events remains low. Gastrointestinal side effects tend to decrease over time as patients adjust.
    - Muscle Preservation: When combined with a high-protein diet and resistance training, studies have shown that lean muscle mass is generally preserved.

- **Quality of Life:** Patients report sustained improvements in daily functioning, energy levels, and overall well-being.
  - **Ongoing Research:** Long-term observational studies continue to monitor cardiovascular outcomes, liver function, and other metabolic parameters to ensure the safety of prolonged use.

Evidence-Based Outcomes

- **Weight Loss Data:** Across multiple trials, GLP-1 therapies have consistently delivered significant weight loss (typically in the range of 10–20% of baseline weight), which is a remarkable achievement compared to traditional interventions.
- **Metabolic Benefits:** Reductions in HbA1c levels, improvements in blood pressure, and favorable shifts in lipid profiles have been documented, suggesting comprehensive metabolic benefits.
- **Quality of Life Enhancements:** Improvements in physical mobility, self-esteem, and psychosocial outcomes have been noted in patient-reported outcomes.
- **Safety Profile:** The majority of adverse events are mild to moderate in severity and tend to resolve over time, affirming the favorable risk–benefit ratio of these therapies.

In Conclusion, the robust body of evidence from major clinical trials underscores the transformative potential of GLP-1 therapies in the management of obesity and metabolic disorders. As ongoing research continues to refine our understanding, these treatments not only deliver significant weight loss but also improve metabolic health and quality of life. This evidence-based approach is critical for both clinicians and patients when considering GLP-1 medications as part of a comprehensive weight management strategy.

Conclusion
Understanding the Complexity of Weight Loss

The Multifaceted Nature of Weight Loss

In the expansive journey of understanding weight loss, physiological aspects stand as a foundational pillar. The body's metabolism plays a crucial role in this process, often acting as the gatekeeper to how efficiently we convert food into energy and manage weight.

For many, metabolism can be enigmatic — some individuals seem to burn calories effortlessly, while others struggle despite similar efforts.

This variance can often be attributed to genetic predispositions. Certain genes influence our metabolic rate, dictating whether we are inclined to gain or lose weight easily.

Hormonal influences such as those from the thyroid gland, insulin levels, and stress hormones like cortisol are pivotal. They regulate how our bodies store fat, utilize energy, and respond to dietary intake.

Understanding these elements provides insights into why a one-size-fits-all approach to dieting rarely works.

Moving beyond the physical, psychological dimensions impact weight management deeply and subtly. Our brains govern not just what we eat, but why we eat.

Cognitive behaviors, including habits like mindless snacking or portion sizes, play significant roles in weight loss efforts. Emotional eating patterns are particularly pervasive; food is often a comfort during stress, sadness, or even boredom. Mental health challenges, such as anxiety or depression, further complicate this landscape, often creating barriers to healthy eating patterns.

It's crucial to recognize these emotional and cognitive triggers and address them in any comprehensive weight loss strategy.

Strategies like mindful eating, behavioral therapy, and supportive environments can create healthier relationships with food and contribute positively to enduring lifestyle changes.

Society adds another layer of complexity. Cultural norms and societal pressures heavily influence perceptions of body image, which can dictate dieting trends and individual behaviors. These pressures manifest in myriad ways — through the media, peer influence, and social expectations, all of which can lead to unrealistic beauty standards and unhealthy dieting practices like crash diets or extreme restrictions.

In some cultures, larger body sizes are historically associated with wealth and health, whereas others celebrate thinness. The battle against obesity stigma involves recognizing these biases and understanding that successful weight management looks different for everyone. Encouraging acceptance of diverse body shapes and promoting health over aesthetics can liberate individuals from the shackles of unrealistic societal expectations.

Every person's path to weight loss is unique, shaped by individualized journeys that account for distinct lifestyle habits, personal motivations, and environmental influences. Lifestyle habits, such as active versus sedentary routines, significantly influence weight outcomes.

Someone with an active lifestyle may naturally have healthier weight management compared to someone who spends most of their day sitting.

Personal motivations also vary; while some embark on this journey for health reasons, others might be driven by self-esteem or external validation. Environmental influences, such as accessibility to healthy food options, poverty, and community support, further shape one's weight management journey.

Tailoring weight loss approaches to accommodate these individual factors is essential for success. Personalized nutrition counseling, flexible exercise plans, and inclusive support systems like group classes or online communities can help sustain motivation and drive results.

Recognizing and respecting these unique pathways foster sustainable change, ensuring that weight loss is achievable and maintained in a holistic manner.

Role of GLP-1 Medications in Weight Management

In the exploration of weight loss, GLP-1 medications emerge as a significant player, offering an innovative approach to managing body weight. These medications, based on the activity of Glucagon-Like Peptide-1, are designed to mimic natural hormones that play crucial roles in appetite regulation.

By doing so, they help individuals feel fuller after eating by signaling fullness and satiety to the brain, thereby reducing the urge to eat more than necessary. This mechanism taps into the body's natural pathways, allowing users to manage their food intake effectively without feeling deprived, which is often a challenge in conventional dieting.

Beyond appetite regulation, GLP-1 medications have a profound impact on metabolic functions. One of the key areas where they excel is in lowering blood sugar levels. For many, particularly those struggling with Type 2 diabetes or insulin resistance, maintaining stable blood sugar is imperative for overall health and effective weight management. Improved blood sugar levels can lead to enhanced energy use within the body, preventing excess sugar from being stored as fat.

However, it's important to understand that while these medications provide substantial benefits, they cannot alone shoulder the responsibility of weight loss. Instead, they should be viewed as supportive aids within a broader strategy, that includes lifestyle interventions such as diet and exercise.

For instance, combining GLP-1 medications with a balanced protein-rich diet with whole foods, not only reinforces calorie control, but also ensures nutrient adequacy, which is essential in any weight loss journey.

Similarly, incorporating regular physical activity helps amplify the benefits of GLP-1 medications by boosting metabolic rate and promoting cardiovascular health.

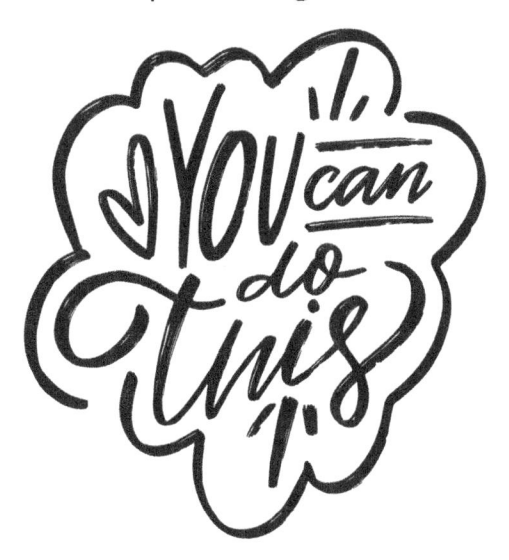

Low-Carb High-Protein Recipes

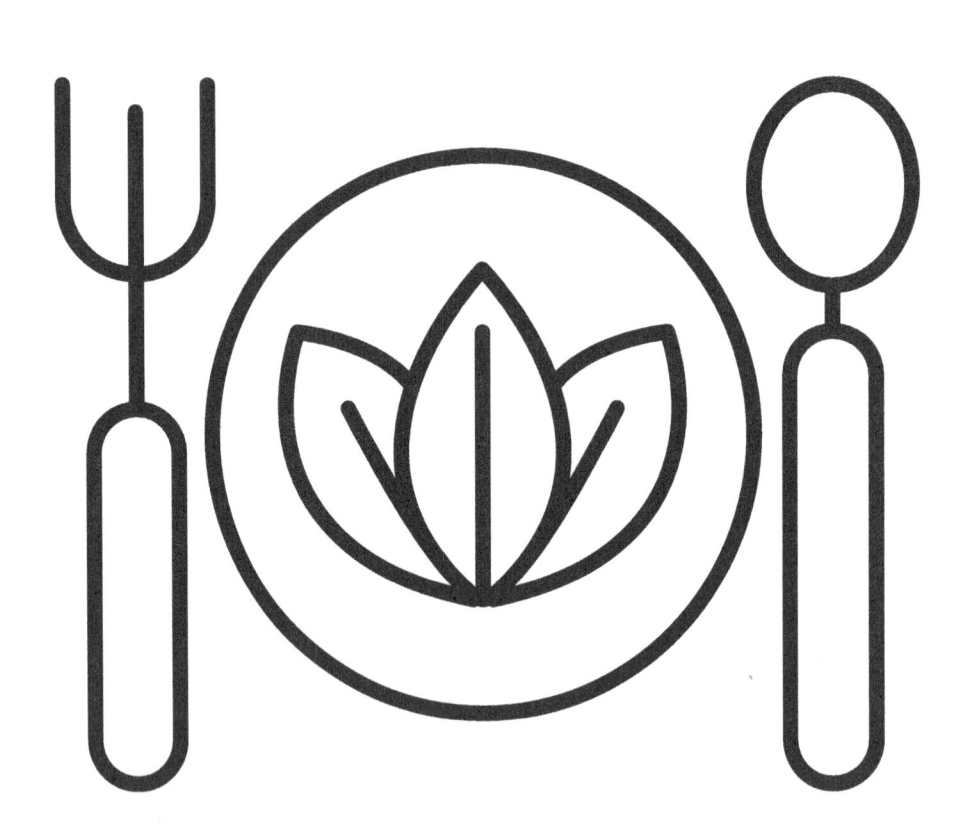

LOW CARB PROTEIN WAFFLES

Ingredients:
- 1 scoop of QUEST protein powder (I like the Peanut Butter or Cinnamon Crunch flavors, but it's your choice which flavor you prefer. It also does not have to be the Quest brand.
- 1 tablespoon of Sour Cream
- 1 Large Egg
- 2 Tablespoons Unsweetened Almond Milk (or Heavy Whipping Cream)
- 1 Teaspoon of Baking Powder
- Pinch of Cinnamon (optional)
- Optional Toppings: Berries, Sugar-Free Syrup, Real Butter (made from sweet cream, not oil), or "No Sugar Added PB Fit" peanut butter powder (with enough water added to it, to make it like a syrup you can drizzle on top)

Instructions:
1. In a bowl, mix together the protein powder, baking powder and Cinnamon.
2. Add in your egg, sour cream, & almond milk/cream, mix well until smooth. No lumps.
3. Heat up your waffle iron and spray it with an olive oil or avocado oil cooking spray.
4. Pour your batter onto the hot waffle iron, and cook until the waffle is golden brown, as desired. This usually takes 3 or 4 minutes max.
5. Remove from waffle iron & add your desired topping.
(Eat with some Bacon or Sausage on the side, and Enjoy! Makes enough for one person to eat)

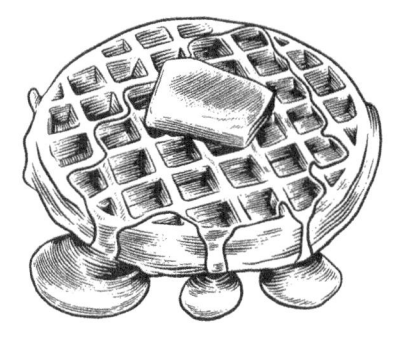

CHEESY EGG MUFFINS

Ingredients:
- Shredded Cheese (your choice - Coby Jack, Cheddar, Mozzarela)
- Chives (or chopped Green Onions, or whatever type of Onions your prefer. Maybe you don't want any)
- Diced Cherry Tomatoes
- 2 or 3 Large Eggs
- Spices - a little Salt, Pepper, & Garlic Powder

Instructions:
1. Pre-Heat Oven to 400 F
2. Get a Muffin pan out. Add muffin foils/papers into the pan & lightly spray them with olive or avocado oil.
3. In a small bowl, mix all the ingredients & spices together.
4. Pour into the muffin pan accordingly, and bake for 10 to 15 minutes. (Or until a "Toothpick Test" comes out clean)
5. Remove from oven & let cool for a few minute. Then eat & enjoy!

Side Note: Eggs will be your best friend on this diet! I eat eggs in every way they can be made. Egg Muffins, Scrambled eggs (chopped up or kept whole as an omlet), Fried Eggs, Poached Eggs, Hard Boiled Eggs... This past Thanksgiving - I ate some Ham, a couple "Deviled Eggs" and a a serving-spoon/scoop of cheesy Broccoli.
I got full, I felt satisfied... Did not feel the need to cheat at all...
It was awesome. But my point is, become BFFs with eggs lol!

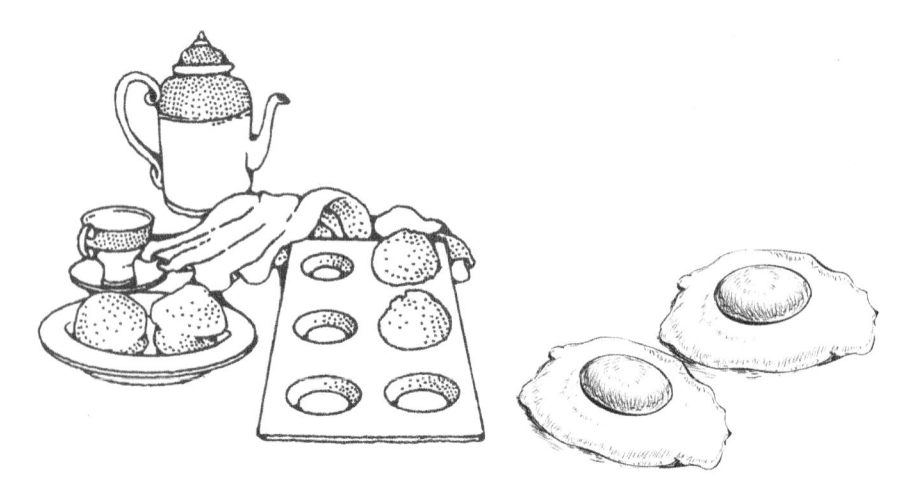

Eggplant & Bacon Alfredo
My Favorite Pasta Replacement

Ingredients:

- 1 pound Bacon
- 1 Cup Heavy Whipping Cream
- 2 tablespoons Butter (real Sweet Cream, not the oil kind)
- 1 tablespoon White Wine
- 1 tablespoon Lemon Juice
- 1 cup Shredded Parmesan Cheese
- Spices - Onion Powder, Garlic Powder, Salt, Pepper, & Parsley

Instructions:

1. Chop up the bacon and fry over medium heat in a large skillet.
2. When the bacon has rendered out and becomes crisp then remove it from the pan, and drain on paper towels. Save all of the bacon grease in the pan/skill et. Crush cooled bacon into bits!
3. Peel & cut the eggplant into pieces the size/shape similar to penne pasta. Cook it in the bacon grease until it softens.
4. The eggplant with soak up the bacon grease as it's cooking, making it soft & more pasta-textured. Add in 2 tablespoons of butter, and mix the melted butter all over the eggplant "pasta"...
5. Pour the cup of heavy whipping cream into the pan. Add the white wine & lemon juice, and stir together... Add your spices! And then add in your shredded parmesan cheese. Stir/Mix!
6. Mix in half of the bacon bits, while finishing up the last couple minutes of it cooking. And use the other half of the bacon bits to sprinkle on top, once on a plate to serve.

And Enjoy!

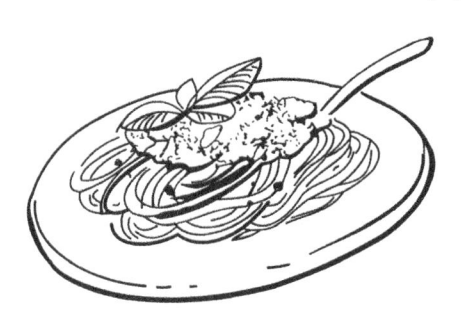

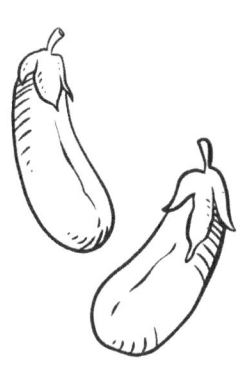

LOW CARB NACHOS

Ingredients:

- Pork Rinds (or small bag of Quest Protein Chips in the Taco flavor)
- Handful of "Mexican Blend" shredded cheese You choice of low carb Salsa (check nutrition label on back of jar)
- Optional: Sour Cream, low carb guacamole, and/or Green Chilis
- Add Protein by cooking some shredded chicken or ground beef beforehand. This is Optional!

Instructions:

1. In a small bowl, add your pork rinds or protein chips. Sprinkle a Handful of shredded cheese on top.
2. Microwave for 30 seconds at a time, keeping a close eye on the cheese. Only microwave long enough to melt the cheese.

Side Note: If you made chicken or ground beef beforehand, use it while it's hot enoughto melt the cheese itself, as to avoid the microwave. Because the Microwave can mess the chips up, if accidently done too long...

3. Once Cheese is melted, add your other low carb toppings & Enjoy!

Prior to weight loss, nachos was one of my favorite comfort foods to munch on. Creating a low carb, high protein way to continue having nachos was a nice way to stay on track. This is an example of how you can still enjoy foods that would not normally be diet friendly, as long as you use the right ingredients to substitute the bad kind!

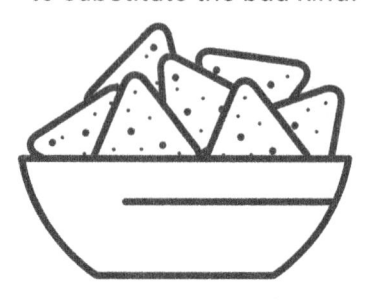

Garlic Parmesan Crusted Chicken

Ingredients:
- 2 boneless, skinless chicken breasts
- ½ cup grated Parmesan cheese
- ¼ cup almond flour (or crushed pork rinds for extra crunch)
- 1 tsp garlic powder
- ½ tsp paprika
- ½ tsp salt
- ¼ tsp black pepper
- 1 large egg
- 1 tbsp olive oil or butter

Instructions:
1. Preheat oven to 400°F (200°C) and line a baking sheet with parchment paper.
2. Flatten chicken breasts slightly for even cooking (optional).
3. Prepare coating: In a shallow bowl, mix Parmesan, almond flour, garlic powder, paprika, salt, and pepper.
4. Beat the egg in a separate bowl.
5. Dip each chicken breast in the egg, then coat with the Parmesan mixture, pressing to adhere.
6. Heat olive oil in a skillet over medium heat. Sear the chicken for 2-3 minutes per side until golden.
7. Transfer to baking sheet and bake for 12-15 minutes or until cooked through (internal temp: 165°F/74°C).
8. Let rest for 5 minutes, then serve!

Serving Ideas:
- Pair with roasted broccoli or a side of cauliflower mash for a balanced low-carb meal.
- Drizzle with sugar-free marinara for an Italian twist.

Baked Salmon with Asparagus and Lemon Butter

Ingredients:

- 2 salmon fillets (about 6 ounces each)
- 1 bunch asparagus, trimmed
- 1-2 tablespoons olive oil
- Salt and pepper, to taste 2 cloves garlic, minced

For the Lemon Butter Sauce:

- 2 tablespoons unsalted butter
- Juice of 1/2 lemon
- 1 tablespoon fresh parsley, chopped
- Optional: a pinch of red pepper flakes for a little heat

Instructions:

1. Preheat your oven to 400°F (200°C). Line a baking sheet with parchment paper or lightly grease it.
2. Place the salmon fillets in the center of the baking sheet. Arrange the asparagus around the salmon. Drizzle olive oil over the salmon and asparagus, then sprinkle the garlic, salt, and pepper evenly over both.
3. Bake in the preheated oven for 12–15 minutes, or until the salmon is cooked through (it should flake easily with a fork) and the asparagus is tender.
4. While the salmon and asparagus are baking, prepare the lemon butter sauce in a small saucepan over low heat. Melt the butter, stir in the lemon juice, chopped parsley, and red pepper flakes (if using), then remove from heat.
5. Once ready, plate the salmon and asparagus, then drizzle the lemon butter sauce over the top. This dish pairs well with a light side salad or steamed broccoli for an extra boost of greens.

AIR FRIED/SKILLET FRIED SALMON PATTIES

Ingredients:

- 1 or 2 small drained cans of skinless/boneless wild-caught
- Salmon
- Diced white/yellow Onions
- Finely Chopped Bell Pepper
- 1 or 2 Handfuls of Unflavored Pork Rinds, Crushed into Crumbs
- 1 Large Egg 1 tablespoon
- Mayo & Spices - Salt, Pepper, & Garlic Powder

Instructions:

1. In a bowl, mix together the Salmon, Onions, & Bell Pepper
2. After Mixed, carefully drain any remaining excess water from the bowl into the sink, without spilling your ingredients.
3. Once that's done, you can add the remaining ingredients. One large egg, mayo, spices, and crushed pork rinds.
4. Once mixed well, you can use either an air fryer, or skillet/frying pan... Lightly Spray air fryer, or pour enoung olive/avocado oil into a pan, to cook patties.
5. Use your hands to form rounded Salmon Patties. They will look like thick "Burger Patties" in shape.
6. Add into skillet or air fryer, and cook until both sides are golded brown.

Be gentle, they do like to crumble apart. But they are worth it! They taste amazing! I like to add some "No Sugar Added" ketchup on top of mine. Fish are another best friend on this diet. Tuna, Salmon, Cod, Shrimp... It just depends how you make it, or what you add to it! But Fish is low carb & high protein (as is all meat)

Buffalo Chicken Stuffed Peppers

Spicy, cheesy, and packed with protein!

Ingredients:

- 2 large bell peppers, halved and seeds removed
- 2 cups shredded cooked chicken (rotisserie chicken works great!)
- ½ cup Greek yogurt
- ¼ cup cream cheese, softened
- ¼ cup buffalo sauce (adjust to taste)
- ½ tsp garlic powder
- ½ tsp onion powder
- ½ cup shredded cheddar or mozzarella cheese 1 tbsp chopped green onions (optional)

Instructions:

1. Preheat oven to 375°F (190°C). Line a baking sheet with parchment paper.
2. Prepare the filling: In a bowl, mix shredded chicken, Greek yogurt, cream cheese, buffalo sauce, garlic powder, and onion powder until well combined.
3. Stuff the peppers: Spoon the buffalo chicken mixture evenly into the halved bell peppers.
4. Top with cheese: Sprinkle shredded cheddar or mozzarella on top.
5. Bake for 20-25 minutes, until the peppers are tender and the cheese is melted and bubbly.
6. Garnish with green onions and serve hot!

Low-Carb Chicken Spaghetti with Spaghetti Squash

A creamy and delicious low-carb alternative to classic chicken spaghetti

Ingredients:

For the Spaghetti Squash:

- 1 medium spaghetti squash
- 1 tbsp olive oil
- ½ tsp salt
- ½ tsp black pepper

For the Chicken & Sauce:

- 2 cups cooked, shredded chicken (rotisserie works well)
- 2 tbsp butter or olive oil
- 3 cloves garlic, minced
- ½ cup diced onion
- ½ cup diced tomatoes (or Rotel for spice)
- 1 cup heavy cream
- ½ cup chicken broth
- ½ cup cream cheese, softened
- 1 tsp Italian seasoning
- ½ tsp paprika
- ½ tsp salt (adjust to taste)
- ¼ tsp black pepper
- ½ cup shredded cheddar cheese
- ½ cup shredded mozzarella cheese

Instructions:

Step 1: Roast the Spaghetti Squash

1. Preheat oven to 400°F (200°C).
2. Cut the spaghetti squash in half lengthwise and remove the seeds.
3. Brush the inside with olive oil, sprinkle with salt and pepper, and place cut side down on a baking sheet.

Continued on Next Page

Low-Carb Chicken Spaghetti with Spaghetti Squash
(continued)

4. Roast for 30-40 minutes, until the squash is tender and can be shredded with a fork.
5. Let cool slightly, then scrape out the spaghetti-like strands with a fork and set aside.

Step 2: Make the Creamy Chicken Sauce

6. In a large skillet, melt butter over medium heat. Add garlic and onion, sautéing for 2-3 minutes until fragrant.
7. Stir in diced tomatoes and cook for another minute.
8. Pour in heavy cream and chicken broth, then add cream cheese. Stir until smooth and combined.
9. Season with Italian seasoning, paprika, salt, and pepper.
10. Add shredded chicken and let simmer for 5 minutes, allowing the flavors to blend.

Step 3: Assemble & Bake

11. Stir the cooked spaghetti squash into the sauce until well coated.
12. Transfer everything into a baking dish, top with cheddar and mozzarella cheese.
13. Bake at 375°F (190°C) for 10-15 minutes, until the cheese is melted and bubbly.
14. Let cool for a few minutes, then serve hot!

Optional Garnishes:
Fresh parsley or basil
Crushed red pepper flakes for heat

Chocolate Avocado Mousse

A rich, creamy dessert packed with healthy fats and protein!

Ingredients:

- 1 ripe avocado
- 2 tbsp unsweetened cocoa powder
- 1 scoop chocolate or vanilla protein powder
- 2 tbsp almond milk (or more for desired consistency)
- 1 tbsp sugar-free sweetener (like stevia or monk fruit)
- ½ tsp vanilla extract
- A pinch of sea salt

Instructions:

1. Blend all ingredients in a food processor or blender until smooth and Creamy.
2. Adjust thickness by adding more almond milk if needed.
3. Taste and adjust sweetness if desired.
4. Chill for 15-30 minutes in the fridge for best texture.
5. Serve with a sprinkle of cocoa powder or berries on top.

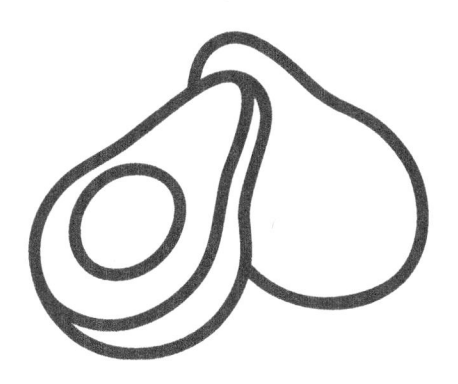

Peanut Butter Chocolate Protein Brownies

Ingredients

- 1 cup natural, unsweetened peanut butter
- 1/3 cup unsweetened cocoa powder
- 3 large eggs
- 1/4 cup unsweetened almond milk
- 1/2 cup keto-friendly sweetener (like erythritol; adjust to taste)
- 1 scoop chocolate (or unflavored) whey protein isolate
- 1/2 tsp baking powder
- 1 tsp vanilla extract
- A pinch of salt
- Optional: A handful of chopped peanuts or sugar-free chocolate chips

Instructions

1. Prep the Oven: Preheat the oven to 350°F (175°C). Line an 8×8-inch baking pan with parchment paper.
2. Mix the Wet Ingredients: In a bowl, whisk together the eggs, almond milk, peanut butter, sweetener, and vanilla extract until smooth.
3. Combine Dry Ingredients: Sift in the cocoa powder, whey protein, baking powder, and salt. Stir until just combined. If you're using optional add-ins (like chopped peanuts or sugar-free chocolate chips), fold them in gently.
4. Bake: Pour the batter into the prepared pan and smooth the top. Bake for 20–25 minutes, or until a toothpick inserted in the center comes out mostly clean.
5. Cool & Cut: Allow the brownies to cool completely in the pan before cutting into squares.

No-Bake Keto Cheesecake

Ingredients
For the Crust

- 1 1/2 cups almond flour
- 3 tbsp unsalted butter, melted
- 2 tbsp keto-friendly sweetener (such as erythritol or monk fruit)
- A pinch of salt

For the Filling

- 16 oz (2 packages) cream cheese, softened
- 1/2 cup sour cream (or Greek yogurt for an extra protein boost)
- 1/3 cup keto-friendly sweetener (adjust to taste)
- 1 tsp vanilla extract
- Juice of 1/2 lemon (optional, for a subtle tang)
- 1/2 cup heavy cream, whipped to stiff peaks
- Optional: 1 scoop unflavored whey protein isolate (for additional protein)

Instructions

1. **Prepare the Crust:**
   - In a medium bowl, mix together the almond flour, melted butter, sweetener, and salt until well combined.
   - Press the mixture firmly into the bottom of a 9-inch springform pan (or any small cheesecake pan) to form an even base.
   - Place the pan in the refrigerator while you prepare the filling to help set the crust.

Continued on Next Page

No-Bake Keto Cheesecake (continued)

1. **Make the Filling:**
   - In a large mixing bowl, beat the softened cream cheese until smooth and creamy.
   - Add the sour cream, keto-friendly sweetener, vanilla extract, and lemon juice (if using), then beat until fully combined.
   - If you're adding whey protein for an extra protein boost, blend it in at this stage until well incorporated.
   - Gently fold in the whipped heavy cream until the mixture is light and smooth. This step helps achieve a silky, mousse-like texture.
2. **Assemble & Chill:**
   - Pour the filling over the chilled crust, smoothing the top with a spatula for an even layer.
   - Cover the pan and refrigerate for at least 4 hours, or overnight, until the cheesecake is firm and set.
3. **Serve:**
   - Once set, remove the cheesecake from the pan and slice into wedges.
   - Enjoy it as is or garnish with a few keto-friendly berries, a dusting of cocoa powder, or sugar-free chocolate shavings for an extra touch.

~ Common Kitchen Swaps ~
Your Ultimate Guide to Low-Carb High-Protein Alternatives

Flour & Baking Alternatives
- Almond Flour: A popular low-carb substitute for wheat flour; it also adds a modest amount of protein and healthy fats.
- Coconut Flour: Extremely low in carbs and high in fiber. Use in combination with other flours for better texture.
- Flaxseed Meal: Provides fiber, omega-3s, and a bit of protein; great for binding in baked goods.

Dairy & Egg Swaps
- Full-Fat Greek Yogurt: High in protein and lower in carbs than regular yogurt—ideal for dressings, dips, or as a base for smoothies.
- Cottage Cheese (Full-Fat): A protein-packed alternative that works well in both savory and sweet recipes.
- Eggs: A versatile, high-quality protein source that can replace higher-carb items in many dishes.

Protein Boosters
- Whey Protein Isolate: Adds a significant protein boost with minimal carbs—perfect for shakes, desserts, and baked goods.
- Collagen Peptides: Easily dissolvable in liquids, these are nearly carb-free and support joint and skin health.
- Plant-Based Protein Powder: Options like pea protein can be used in recipes where you want to boost protein without dairy.

(Continued on Next Page)

Common Kitchen Swaps Continued

Pasta, Rice & Grain Substitutes

- Zucchini Noodles (Zoodles): A low-carb alternative to traditional pasta with a fresh, light texture.
- Shirataki Noodles: Made from konjac yam, these noodles are nearly carb-free and calorie-free, making them a great pasta substitute.
- Cauliflower Rice: Use grated or processed cauliflower as a substitute for rice in stir-fries, bowls, or side dishes.

Vegetable-Based Alternatives

- Spaghetti Squash: When roasted, its strands mimic pasta, offering a low-carb base for sauces and other toppings.
- Mashed Cauliflower: A creamy, low-carb replacement for mashed potatoes, often enriched with butter or cream cheese for extra protein.

Nuts, Seeds & Butters

- Nuts & Seeds (e.g., almonds, walnuts, chia seeds): They offer healthy fats and protein. Use them whole, chopped, or ground for a crunchy texture in recipes.
- Nut Butters (Almond, Peanut Butter – unsweetened): Great for adding flavor, protein, and healthy fats to smoothies, sauces, or baked goods.
- Cheese: Varieties like cheddar, mozzarella, and cream cheese are not only low in carbs but also pack a good protein punch, making them excellent in sauces, salads, or as toppings.

Two Worthy Mentions

- Nutritional Yeast (has B vitamins & a little protein. Taste like Cheese)
- Pork Rinds (can be crushed and used to substitute crackers as a binding agent in meatloaf or salmon patties. Or as a crunchy coating/crust on meats like chicken)

Thank You

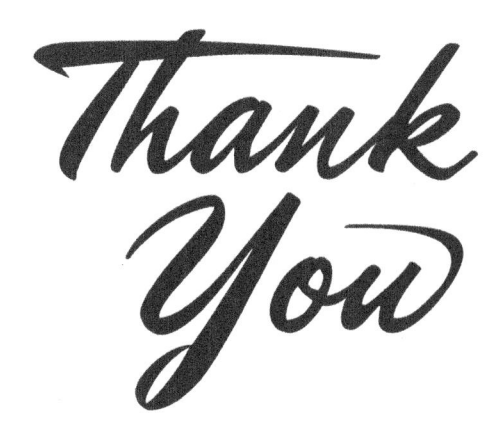

For reading "The GLP-1 Advantage: Beyond the Injections"

If you Found this Book Helpful,
Leaving a **Review** would be Greatly Appreciated.
Good Luck on your Journey!

Brittany Alana

weight tracker

STARTING WEIGHT   **GOAL WEIGHT**

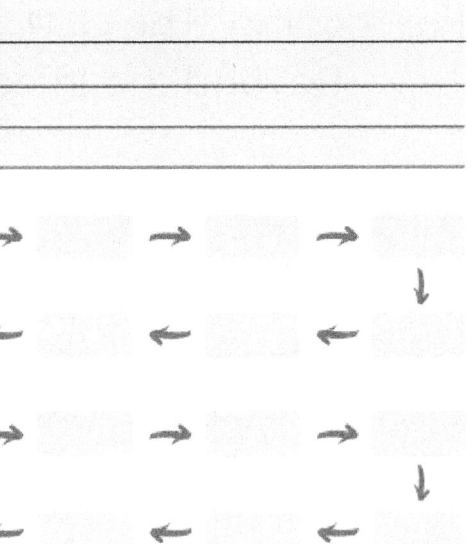

NOTES

_____
_____
_____

Personal Notes

Personal Notes